Unfrosted

Get <u>Real</u> About Food and Fitness

No Sugarcoating

Raven Grimaldi

Disclaimer

The opinions expressed in this book are entirely my own, drawn from personal experience, observation, research and common sense. This book is not designed to offend anyone, but it probably will anyway. It's not politically correct, for the overly sensitive or those in denial. If you're part of the food or diet industry, you already know the truth. If you're overweight, (and I'm talking anybody who has muffin-top above wherever the waistline on your jeans might be when you sit – come on, don't play dumb) it's way past time you owned up to it and by virtue of the fact that you're reading this, maybe you're there. So be honest with yourself, laugh, and plunge on.

Don't attempt any of the diet modifications or exercise suggestions in this book without first checking with a medical professional. I know you're going to do this.

Table of Contents

Preface

It's a roller coaster, isn't it? Maybe as though you were stuck in some fairy tale where no matter how hard you try, the wicked witch cackles when you step on the scales. For some reason, the weight comes back. Sometimes, it's just five or ten pounds. So, to get ready for the New Year's Eve party because you bought that dress with gold sequins three months ago that you knew you'd be able to get into by then, you literally starve for four days and wear it with a body shaper, hoping you won't get tipsy on the first glass of wine because you haven't eaten all day, and frankly, you're afraid to go near the buffet at all.

After a few years of this, the scales betray you again and it's ten or twenty pounds. You adjust, buy the size 10 or 12 or 14 and hate designers who even say the words "size 0 or 2". You don't look fat, exactly, just not like a model anymore, or that teenage girl you saw in Macy's Saturday trying on Lucky jeans that actually fit her. You start buying T-shirts that have a little room over the waistband instead of the spandex ones, in case you want to sit down and not have the fat roll show.

Maybe it's a lot more than twenty pounds, and you're having trouble getting around like you used to, and have given up doing a lot of the things you enjoyed because it's just too hard anymore. Perhaps your doctor has put you on a recommended diet, or some medications for high blood pressure, or stomach problems, or mild depression. It could get worse from there.

If any of this sounds at all familiar, get real. The book cover didn't lie. No more sugarcoating: not with your food, and not with what you're about to read. I'm going to tell you how it is, and how you can take charge and fix it. I know, it sounds tough, but I care. Email me and let me know how you're doing: ravengrimaldi@gmail.com.

Preface

It's a roller coaster, isn't it? Maybe as though you were stuck in some fairy tale where no matter how hard you try, the wicked witch cackles when you step on the scales. For some reason, the weight comes back. Sometimes, it's just five or ten pounds. So, to get ready for the New Year's Eve party because you bought that dress with gold sequins three months ago that you knew you'd be able to get into by then, you literally starve for four days and wear it with a body shaper, hoping you won't get tipsy on the first glass of wine because you haven't eaten all day, and frankly, you're afraid to go near the buffet at all.

After a few years of this, the scales betray you again and it's ten or twenty pounds. You adjust, buy the size 10 or 12 or 14 and hate designers who even say the words "size 0 or 2". You don't look fat, exactly, just not like a model anymore, or that teenage girl you saw in Macy's Saturday trying on Lucky jeans that actually fit her. You start buying T-shirts that have a little room over the waistband instead of the spandex ones, in case you want to sit down and not have the fat roll show.

Maybe it's a lot more than twenty pounds, and you're having trouble getting around like you used to, and have given up doing a lot of the things you enjoyed because it's just too hard anymore. Perhaps your doctor has put you on a recommended diet, or some medications for high blood pressure, or stomach problems, or mild depression. It could get worse from there.

If any of this sounds at all familiar, get real. The book cover didn't lie. No more sugarcoating: not with your food, and not with what you're about to read. I'm going to tell you how it is, and how you can take charge and fix it. I know, it sounds tough, but I care. Email me and let me know how you're doing: ravengrimaldi@gmail.com.

Chapter One
The Beginning of the End

You're jaded. You're disappointed, frustrated, burned out, and tired of wasting money. You don't want to hear any more hysterical commercials with has-been TV actresses who shrilly proclaim how much weight they've lost on some wonderful program or buy another diet book by a doctor (whose specialty might be pathology for all you know) who discovered that eating raw turnips, rare steak, running four miles a day and drinking green tea at 4 AM by the light of the setting moon is the secret to weight loss, and quite possibly, immortality.

That's why I wrote this book – to tell the truth about dieting, weight loss and the food we eat. When I say this is the best food, diet and workout advice that's ever been written down, and you're about to embark on a life-changing journey, not just for you, but probably everyone you live with, you may not believe me at first. That's a pretty sweeping statement to make. I don't have a TV show, I didn't used to be a model, I'm not selling special food, equipment, power bars, vitamins, recipe plans, and I don't even have a website to promote myself. How can I be trusted if I'm not going to make big money off your misery? That's practically un-American.

It's also the reason you can trust me.

You know how the weight loss and diet industry works, because you see it in magazines and on TV every day:

- Jenny Craig Weight Loss with the indomitable Kirstie Alley (she's still fat but make-up, lighting and marketing are wonderful things) pay up and enjoy their "food"

- Weight Watchers – the endless meetings, the "Points", the calculating and processed frozen dinners, if you want to buy them

- L. A. Weight Loss – more money and more processed food

- Slim Fast – yeah, shakes and bars until you don't ever want to hear those words again

- NutriSystem – pay up again and more "food"

- Herbal wonder pills and formulas – these never really work and your blood pressure can go nuts because some of the herbs are supposed to speed your metabolism up and can have some side effects

- Infomercials that have a plethora of people who will assure you that if you pay your money you can look like them but you won't, and besides, Calista Flockhart looks like she's ready for the grave in real life, Harrison Ford aside.

- Calorie-counting, food-exchanging, weighing portions

You also see it in the supermarket every time you check out, and I know that when you're standing in line, you riffle through the magazines, because at least half of the ones on the rack (conveniently placed for your reading pleasure, hey thanks, Safeway) have cover stories that always include "Gourmet Meals in 10 Minutes", "Desserts Like Grandma's for the Busy

Woman", and right there with the junk food, "Lose 20 Pounds in a Month", or "New Miracle Seasoning that Melts Off Pounds" or my personal favorite: "Have a Bikini Body by Beach Time." (These usually start showing up in March and run through June, so they're giving you blunder time here.)

OK, you're not going to be taken in by this crap. You're intelligent and well-read, so you snort with disdain and go to the bookstore. You've bought a lot of books about this very thing, and were really enthusiastic for a few weeks after you read each one, recommending them to your friends, your family and you followed the advice:

- The Sonoma Diet

- The South Beach Diet

- Ultrametabolism

- Ten Years Younger

- Dr. Pritikin's Diet

- Dr. Atkins Diet

- Sooo many others

There's a new one every day, a best-seller every month. Seems like every MD or waning movie star who's ever thought about making a quick buck has penned a diet opus. Check the New York Times lists if you don't believe me. Everybody wants a healthier, slimmer body because they know they need to "treat their body as a temple," only put healthy foods into it, slim down, live longer, not have a heart attack, lower their cholesterol.

What you also want is to be hot. The rest of it is window dressing. Let's get real. Fortunately for you, if you get out of denial and do what I suggest, you will also:

- Get rid of the fat

- Lower your cholesterol

- Lower your blood pressure

- Feel great instead of tired

- Have better skin and shiny hair

- Live longer

- Get out of bed every morning and like what you see in the mirror

- Have fun buying clothes that look good on you instead of worrying about covering up the muffin-top above your waistband

- Breathe more easily

- Be able to run if you have to, possibly even four blocks at a dead heat

- Laugh more

- Wear something besides black (summer happens everywhere, remember that)

- Have fun, get on with the really important stuff in your life, and really like yourself

Because, "hot" isn't only about how you look, but how you breathe, move, laugh and live your life, and how your eyes sparkle. It's also about what you eat. Remember that old saying: garbage in, garbage out? It should be "garbage in, garbage STAYS." Everything works together.

There's a better way to eat, live and get on with your life, and all this hucksterism is not it. Forget diets, plans, food-exchanging, calorie-counting and listening to anybody who's making money selling you these things. For instance, Nestle Foods, who sell you hundreds of processed food items, including Butterfingers and HotPockets, also owns Jenny Craig. What clever little monkeys they are!

If you bought this book, you need to keep reading it. You also need to do more than just read it. I know, you have the best of intentions. I know this because I've been there myself. I've bought the books and I've read them, I've gone to Target and Amazon and bought the exercise DVDs too. How dusty are those, by the way?

I'm not going to write chapter on chapter about nutrition, body mass indexes, why carbohydrates are evil, how bulgur wheat or cayenne pepper will save your life and melt your fat, case histories about Sherry T. from Long Island and how she turned her life around with my advice, or why corn is hard to digest. I am going to tell you the truth, and how to eat right and get healthy. This is Chapter One, and what I'm telling you here is to read on, and why. It's going to go fast, so keep up. Remember two things:

1. Insanity is doing the same thing over and over again, and expecting different results. (Thank you, Einstein.)

2. Neither the diet industry or the food industry is concerned about you getting slim or healthy, they are solely concerned about making money.

Chapter Two
The Yellow Brick Road to Nowhere

Let's get started. We're going to talk about what you've been doing so far. It hasn't been working the way you wanted it to, has it? Let's talk about why.

You've done the "diets" and the "plans". "Plan" sounds suspiciously like you just joined Scientology or are waiting for the mother ship to arrive on Lone Mountain next Tuesday. "Diet" sounds like a dirty word or something you say, like "I'm on a diet, so I can't have that cheeseburger" or "I 'd love to have a piece of Amy's birthday cake, but I'm on a diet" or some other lame ass remark which lets everyone know you're trying to lose weight or don't like the way you look. Forget it.

First of all, you don't need to say anything, ever. Just "No, thanks", is all you ever need to say. Once you state you're on a "diet" or explain in any way, you've put yourself in the situation where you're anxious because now people expect results that you feel obligated to deliver. Never good. Then what happens is, you ate too much at lunch, so once you get home you're going to break out the chips and salsa, have a Dos Equis or two and say to yourself, screw it, I won't have dinner, and it'll all even out. Also never good.

□□□□

So, first let's look at food – the sort of food that lots of diet books and plans suggest. Let's start with breakfast. Most likely it was supposed to be something like:

- Half a grapefruit, and a boiled egg

- Granola with skim milk, and a banana

- Steel cut oats with blackberries. (I especially love this one, it's so practical because steel cut oats take half an hour to cook and really stick up the pot)

- Or, a poached egg on whole wheat toast
  with three blueberries

- Coffee or tea, black

Odds, are, though, it went something like this, especially after a few days: you had two cups of coffee with French Vanilla creamer while you were drying your hair, because you had an early meeting or got up too late to cook this stuff or even get to the cereal; or you stopped at Starbucks and got a latte and later on the guy from accounting stopped by with bagels and you thought, well OK, maybe just a whole wheat one, with lite cream cheese.

Well, moving on to lunch. Since you're active and it's the middle of the day, you can fuel up a bit. True, but on your diet you're probably advised to eat:

- Tuna salad (with a little lite mayonnaise or
  nothing) and a tomato

- Chicken breast and a salad of lettuce with
  some lemon juice

- Two slices of turkey with lettuce wrapped
  in a whole wheat tortilla

- Two hard-boiled eggs, some brown rice and
  a banana

Let's take a minute and talk about how lunch really went after the first blush of enthusiasm waned. At first, you were pumped. This one's really going to work, and it makes so much sense. You've been good – following the menu, chopping veggies, buying those plastic containers, bringing your lunch so you don't give in to the temptation of the cafeteria, fast food, or going out at noon to that new Thai place. Give me a break. This is beyond boring, for one thing.

Realistically, lunch is when things happen – there's catered food at the office and always yummy leftovers even if you weren't at the meeting, there's the going-away lunch for Joan and you couldn't miss that, pot-luck day when people bring in things like their favorite chili-cheese tostadas and you must participate, business lunches at the Metro Grill, where the Chilean sea bass is on special for $18 and the company's picking up the tab, the PTA is getting together at Linda's or lunch with your friends at the chic new café because you haven't gotten together in ages.

You know it's going to happen this way three days out of five and you need to figure this in. Your carefully packed whatever is going to rot in the office refrigerator or be an afterthought in the fridge at home. Believe me, you're never going to be Jonesing for that dry tuna anyway, so who cares?

Well, you will, because not only are you blowing the diet and soon feeling bad about yourself, but you're losing money on the carefully chosen food you shopped for. Yikes, we're talking double-edged sword and more.

□□□□

Let us not forget "snacks". I love this one. Most of these diets advocate snacks bigtime – morning, mid-afternoon, and my favorite: mid-evening. This is because they say they're worried about your blood sugar and also the fact that you've been hoarding chocolate somewhere and might succumb. (It's in your second desk drawer, or behind the brown rice boxes in the kitchen, where the kids never look. You know where.) It doesn't matter, because snacks are for people who need to seriously get a life. What are you, six years old? Americans have been sold "snacks" as something we deserve since we got home from first grade, but the reality is we don't need to eat them.

You don't need the mid-morning snack, you just think you do because you stopped smoking and just got a nasty phone call from corporate about that report you forgot, or the dog just tried to eat all the pansies you planted yesterday. Deal with it, don't eat because it makes you feel better. The mid-afternoon thing is all about your 3:00 slump (everybody gets one, so go talk to your friend down the hall, or take the dog for a walk before the kids get home.)

The evening one is silly. You've been conditioned to think you need to eat if you watch a movie or TV, thanks to the concession folks and the Doritos people. I especially love Hollywood Video whose racks of pop-corn and movie candy are right there at the checkout, making you think you're supposed to eat if you watch a DVD. All those other people are doing it, aren't they? That's part of the entertainment experience, isn't it?

Well, take a good look at the people in the movie theater stuffing in the popcorn or sour jellies (fatties, most of them) or the charmers on the Tostitos ads on TV – usually teenagers who for now have the growth spurt to burn it off, but are just fatties in their 20s waiting to happen, and it will.

Remember this: anything you eat later on in the evening will stay with you and churn in your stomach all night, and end up on your hips. You've been conned, rethink it. Take up knitting. Or art, or bowling. If you have kids, play games – mental or physical, or both. After they go to bed, an adult activity is good. I'm sure you know what some of those are. Snacks – phhffft.

☐☐☐☐

Let's move on to dinner. For some reason, diets always put the biggest meal at the end of the day and I never could figure this one out, because we have little time to work it off. We don't live in Spain, where people take siestas and then stay up half the night. What's even dumber is the chic hour to eat in restaurants or dinner parties is still eight o'clock. Oh please. I think the reason for this is so everyone can get halfway sloshed on a couple of drinks and not really notice that the quality of food they're wolfing down could be mediocre, as their taste buds and growling stomachs are telling them whatever they're putting in their mouths is a blessing at this point.

I'm pretty sure this is a holdover from the 1950s when men wore suits to work and had three hour martini lunches while their wives stayed home and decorated or played cards and ate bridge mix and cheese out of a can with crackers all afternoon. Guys went to work at 9 AM and most women didn't work out of the house at all. The kids got fed early and put to bed early as well.

Given their day, the adults probably weren't hungry until 8 PM, if at all, they weren't very well informed about nutrition and most of them couldn't give a rat's ass about staying in shape. This was the day of girdles and those Jane Russell pointy-tit bras with round stitching that left embedded strap marks on shoulders. Take a look at old Vogue magazines, it's true. But I digress.

Here's what you're probably advised to have for dinner:

- Baked chicken breast with brown rice and broccoli

- An adventuresome stirfry with tofu, snap peas, onion and broccoli

- Small filet mignon with iceberg lettuce salad, sprinkled with lemon juice

- Baked cod, sliced tomatoes, couscous

- Sounds like entrée city, eh? If this is not enough, usually they throw in a dessert sop. It could be something really yummy like:

- Six vanilla wafers topped with a tablespoon of vanilla yogurt and a sprinkle of cinnamon

- Two strawberries dipped in dark chocolate

- A diet brownie made of God knows what, but not sugar and flour

Wowie. That's a satisfying conclusion to your day, isn't it? Aha – things could also go awry here. Maybe you went to happy hour and the folks at Champs Sports Bar don't specialize in kasha and pine nuts. Or you had dinner with a client, or a friend, neither one of which wants to hear about plans and diets. Or you went to the Little League game and the kids won, (or lost) either of which means a trip to Pizza Hut, or maybe because cooking two or three separate dinners again was just too much to contemplate. Or your significant other wants a romantic evening and lobster is on the menu. Once again, we're back to three out of five and counting.

So there you have it, or something close to it. Yes, if you stay on this diet for two weeks you will probably lose some weight. You will also be crabby, feel a little woozy occasionally, maybe start smoking again, have diarrhea and cramps (depending on just how much soy and hummus you ate) and, after all this, eventually start eating the same things you ate before.

It may take a week or two, sometimes even a month, but you will succumb. And, pretty soon, you'll probably gain all the weight back and maybe even a pound or two more. But you'll think you've learned a lot, about some foods and what you shouldn't eat anymore. Now you're smarter, and a whole lot guiltier, too.

It didn't work out the way you wanted it to, did it? Here's why.

You absolutely cannot change the way you've eaten most of your life just because some book, diet plan or TV show tells you this is how it ought to be, because:

- It takes a lot of time and planning that maybe just isn't going to work out.

- You can't imagine never eating things you really love again, and after two weeks or so, you're getting pissed off about it, really. Even the Taco Bell ads are starting to work on you.

- You have lost some weight but you aren't really feeling all that great.

- You aren't enjoying eating anymore.

- You think about killing every skinny blonde you see and you wish Paris Hilton would choke on a mouthful of Chihuahua hair.

- The food they're telling you to eat really tastes awful.

If you've been on Jenny Craig or any other plan that has you buying processed meals, shakes and bars, you:

- Are spending a lot of money on stuff that tastes pretty much like crap, and if you read the labels, is filled with additives, chemicals and other junk you can't spell

- Feel like the Prisoner of Zenda, because now you're completely dependent on somebody else for your sustenance and advice on how to eat it

- Are dreaming about your mom or grandma's fried chicken and apple pie

- Wish Kristie Alley would trip on those long cover-ups she wears and fall on her make-up-caked overpaid face

- Are wondering why you ever bothered to spend money on cookware, not to mention the fancy kitchen

Here's the thing about any diet or plan that real people have to take into consideration: life happens, shit happens, and you change your plans accordingly. Otherwise, you get very miserable very quickly. Miserable isn't going to help you lose weight or anything else. Eating should be fun, and taste good, and every social occasion there is involves food.

I think we've come full circle. Take the books to the nearest used bookstore. You won't need them anymore. You never did anyway. This one, however, you do. Read on.

☐☐☐☐

There's one more thing. It's called "stress eating", or eating to make yourself feel better. This is where chocolate, hidden Twinkies, or "comfort food" come into play. These terms are designed to make you feel as though you deserve the food you're consuming because you didn't get the raise, or you even lost your job; your boyfriend's into someone else (probably a thinner someone else); your husband's out with his secretary; the kids are driving you crazy and General Hospital isn't cutting it; or somebody cut you off in traffic for the tenth time on the way home. These are biggies, but stress type eaters will eat for almost any reason because their moms told them to have a cookie, it'll make it feel better, or some 100 pound girl on TV is eating chocolate ice cream and watching Casablanca because her boyfriend is a jerk. Stress eaters have conditioned themselves to think they'll feel better if they eat something yummy (and most likely full of high fructose corn syrup (everything processed is) and it won't matter. But it will, especially because you're doing it more than just once or twice. If you find yourself doing this more than once a week, this is a pattern and a habit. Break it. This is not comfort, this is self-destructive. You don't deserve to be fat, so quit kidding yourself because getting fatter's the only thing you're getting out of any comfort in this food. I'm only going to say this once, just like most everything else in this book. I'm not Doctor Phil and I'm not going to be nicey-nice about it. You know it's crap, so: knock it off, grow up, and act like the responsible adult you are.

Chapter Three
Truth and Enlightenment

I said this was going to go fast. We've talked about the past, and we're moving on, to the present, and to your future. If you want to lose weight, keep it off, get in shape and like the way you look and feel, you have to do three simple things, and you have to do them for the rest of your life.

- Eat real food

- Eat less of it

- Get off your butt and move

That's it. I told you it was simple. You want it, you have to throw away your preconceptions, your old habits, your fears and insecurities, and trust me when I say not only does this work, it's the beginning of changing not only your body, but the rest of your life. Sounds dramatic, but it's true.

However, the deck's stacked against you and you're about to do battle with your own preconceptions, as well as the processed food industry, the diet industry, and their persuasive allies – the advertising industry, very powerful foes. However, information is power, and power gives you self-control.

We live in a time and place that's made food gathering, growing, processing, cooking and eating the easiest it's ever been for the human race. (Dogs and cats, too, now that I think of it – not much searching for prey going on there, with Kibbles and Bits and Fanci-Feast – what the hell is with cats on silk cushions eating salmon out of champagne glasses – and we think Rome was decadent. Anyway.)

If you want, you can eat every single meal with as little effort as punching numbers on a microwave, pushing down the toaster button, opening a poptop can, stirring in hot water or stopping at the drive-through. It may not be your first choice, or your favorite meal, but you do it anyway, and you've gotten used to it, sadly enough. What's really sad, though, is your body has gotten just as used to it as your mind, and there's some really bad things happening to it. It's not just that your jeans don't fit, it's much worse. That extra fat tissue, especially around the middle of your body, can be the precursor to diabetes, cardiac issues, gastrointestinal problems and many others.

Fast food is just the obvious tip of the iceberg. Food producers and supermarkets are no better, sometimes worse, because 80% more or less of the stuff offered in these huge food warehouses we all shop in every week is processed in some way but we're under the delusion that it's still better than McDonald's. In many cases, it's not. We'll go into this in depth in the next chapter on eating the right food, but supermarkets lead right to the next conundrum – eating less.

▯▯▯▯

We live in a time and place that is extraordinary in its plenty. Never in the history of the world has so much been offered to so many for so little. We can complain about the cost of coffee, or raspberries, or lettuce this month, or that turkeys cost more than last Thanksgiving, yadda yadda. Come on, this is whining at its finest. We live in a country where most of us can go get as much food as we want, really, anytime we want it. There are no restraints on us, except our grocery budgets. Anything that strikes our fancy, we pretty much buy it and eat it. If we don't know how to cook it, we go to the bakery or get take-out. It's always there and it's always open, sometimes open 24 hours.

I'd like to say hunger will find a way, but it's not hunger, it's really just plain pleasure and gluttony. Oh my, that's an ugly word, isn't it? We'll talk lots more about this in Chapter 5.

So, we find that you can eat whatever you want, whenever you want, and as much of it as makes you satisfied and more. That's the world we live in, and frankly, that's pretty cool. I wouldn't want it any other way, and I'm very glad I live right here right now. I'm not a masochist, my gardens don't always turn out very well and there's some nights I'd get down on my knees to thank Hung Far Low's for the best Kung Pao Chicken on earth that I haven't had to do anything for except whip out the Visa card. But there's a price to be paid for this lovely excess.

☐☐☐☐

Because we live in this land of plenty, we've gotten physically soft and lazy. OK, OK, don't get testy. Maybe you work hard all day at your desk, at the store, at the plant, and expend a lot of mental energy, I know I do. Or you chase kids around the house and play chauffeur half the afternoon, and that's hard work, I've done that too. Or you go to school and run from class to class, and that's both mental and physical drudgery at times, believe me I know that as well.

Life is hectic, crazy, frustrating and some days are wonderful and full of accomplishment while others are just plain hell and you wish you had a Star Trek phaser so every other driver on the road home would get vaporized forever so they'd get out of your way, never mind they might have ten kids in that minivan. (In fact, they usually do, and I'm not sure the world wouldn't be a better place...I mean, those kids could turn out to be serial killers anyway, so actually you'd be doing them a favor when you really think about it because their mother never heard of a turn signal so how much could they be learning from her....yeah, I've had those days, too.)

You're using up energy all right, no question about that. But you're also clenching muscles all over your body, from your eyelids to your toes, all day long. You're breathing erratically, sometimes holding it and other times heaving long sighs. You've tensed up, you've been surprised, you've concentrated, and no matter what – you haven't laughed enough. Maybe some, but nowhere near enough. Nobody does, unfortunately.

You need to MOVE. That would be your body, in random patterns, letting go of all that tension. It's the only way. Meditation is nice, but not enough. Sleep is good, but doesn't work for this. Sex is beneficial, but doesn't do much for your shoulders...well I guess it could, but it's even better if there's some muscle there, anyway still not enough because the Kama Sutra isn't an every night deal for most of us. We're not going there now, that's another book.

I'm talking blood – moving it through your body, your veins, your muscles, and it needs you to move the moveable parts to get the job done. It's called….. are you ready? Exercise. Don't throw down the damn book, you knew it was coming. But, it's better than you think, and…..you get a reprieve until Chapter 6.

☐☐☐☐

That's the scenario, my darlings. Like anything that's worth doing, as my grandfather used to say, it's going to take some doing on your part. There is no free lunch. You can't just go along, hoping there will be some medical breakthrough – the "lose weight pill", just pop it in with your vitamins every morning and eat like a shark. (Incidentally, sharks never get fat, because they never stop moving. If they stop moving, they die. Food for thought, so to speak.)

The rest of this book will give you some information, some advice, some tools, and go into each of these three concepts in depth. You are about to become a guerrilla in the war against fat, mediocrity, advertising and groupthink. You can do this, and you're going to find that once you do, you'll never, ever, want to go back. There's an old saying that will resound for you quite soon: once you know, you have a responsibility to act upon that knowledge.

Chapter Four
Food, Glorious Food.
What's Good and Where to Find It

From the Garden of Eden's apples to Grandma's pot roast, food provides and inspires, comforts and nourishes, and is the centerpiece around which nearly every human social occasion flourishes. We spend huge amounts of time planning, shopping for and preparing it – and we love it when it turns out well. However, somewhere in the last fifty years or so, it's begun to go a little differently. Things have changed, and for a while there it seemed to be a good thing. Convenience, choices, convenience, pre-packaged, convenience, frozen, convenience, fast food, convenience, to go, convenience. Well, maybe I overstated that, but the number one reason we don't eat better food is indeed convenience and the opportunity to buy our food already processed to some degree. We've also been brainwashed by the food processing industry and even the muddled and deluded U.S. Dept. of Agriculture, who can't seem to figure out what real food is anymore.

Pretty much the only occasion still left we start sort of from scratch is Thanksgiving. We're not going out and chopping off the turkey's neck and plucking feathers, but that naked goose-pimply twenty-something pound dead fowl is pretty intimidating. (I remember my college roommate forgetting to take the little bag of icky parts out before she put it in the oven and that was not a good thing....). We make stuffing, boil potatoes and even figure out how to make gravy. Sometimes we get adventurous, looking at fresh sweet potatoes, but usually Aunt Jeannie always brings the ones with marshmallows (yuck) so there's no point in getting carried away.

But what about the rest of the year? Most of you cook, I know that. But some of you don't, not really, unless it's pretty simple, for lots of reasons, and good ones at that – you just simply don't have the time, you don't really know how and don't care about learning, or you don't have to. I respect that, but honestly? If you have a cook, lucky you, and you probably also have a personal trainer and aren't reading this anyway, (but you should be). If not, you need to learn how to do a few things around the kitchen, because you need to be independent and be able to feed yourself. This does not mean opening the frozen food carton. This means eating real food, preparing and cooking it from start to finish, the right stuff.

We've all seen the ever-changing food pyramids and the ever-changing daily nutritional requirements from the U.S. government. In the last few years, they've finally woken up and discovered what most of the world already knew: Americans eat far too much meat and too many dairy products. But the biggest difference in American food in the last 50 years is that we eat industrialized processed food, from feedlot beef to instant dinners.

America is the land of plenty, and plenty of food is what we've been sold, by the government and the food industry. We thought we needed to produce lots of food cheaply, and by God, we did just that. We figured out how to grow lots of corn, soybeans, wheat and rice and process it into tasty boxes and snacks. We put animals in feedlots and factory farms, growing them bigger more quickly, with plenty of hormones and of course plenty of antibiotics to keep them standing up until they were fat enough to slaughter. We eat processed and/or frozen instant breakfasts, lunches and dinners and snacks, snacks, snacks, all chockfull of sugars and chemicals. This is why today, many people:

- Are overweight

- have high cholesterol, high blood pressure, diabetes, heart disease, possibly cancer, acid reflux, gerds and a host of other diseases and symptoms that keep doctors busy and wealthy

- watch and mostly believe pharmaceutical companies' prettily produced advertise-ments that make up a huge segment of the evening's TV fare, touting everything from "bloat" to allergies to men's flagging libido sex aids (You know the ones – some moron lasciviously pops a pill to get lucky later watching his wife bat her eyelashes and try on designer clothes). Here I have to men-tion the latest heavily advertised pharma-ceutical diet pill miracle, available over the counter. People have gone nuts over this stuff, creating a monument to the gullibility and desperation of the American dieter. What a wonderful thing – the cost for these pills averages $2 a day, and I wish I owned stock in Pampers because this drug is a party in your pants, literally. A little reading of the literature that accompanies the pills says:

"While no one likes experiencing treatment effects, they might help you think twice about eating questionable fat content". They aren't kidding with these threats.

"Treatment effects" are what they term loose stools, spotty gas and hard to control bowel movements, which is what happens if people take this drug and don't eat like Gandhi. Here's the real deal: You spend $2 a day to take a drug that gives you uncontrollable diarrhea, (they actually recommend you wear dark clothes and even carry a spare set – hey thanks for the fashion tip, but I think your dancing days are done if you're on this drug), and very likely doesn't help you lose any more weight than you would have on any diet, except for of course having diarrhea all the time. This surpasses just clever marketing, it's just downright scary that anybody would willingly make this choice.

It's time to stop being a victim of the pharmaceutical, weight loss, processed and fast food industry and its advertising and take charge of your diet, two thirds of which should be unprocessed vegetables, fruit and good grains. Period. I don't care what your mom said or what you grew up eating. Start eating real food. No more fast food, boxed quickie dinners, or frozen entrees. No more processed food, period. If you decide to be a vegetarian, even better, but most of us won't, so let's get real. Morton's Steakhouse knows us too well and they aren't worried. Now, since we aren't going out to eat every day, where does the right food come from?

☐☐☐☐

As Michael Pollan so aptly demonstrated in his book "The Omnivore's Dilemma", there's four basic approaches and places to get food:

- Fast food – quick, sometimes tasty, made of the cheapest ingredients, processed in ways and with stuff you don't want to think about, and filled with salt, fat and sugar. Yeah, I know McDonald's has salads since the movie "Supersize Me" embarrassed them, but watch out for the dressings and how long has the lettuce been sitting there?

- The supermarket, where most people shop, which has it all, nearly

- Organic markets, i.e., Whole Foods, Sprouts, Trader Joe's, Pike Place Market in Seattle (miss you!) and hundreds of others around the country: ethnic markets, bakeries, Saturday markets where farmers set up and sell their produce (along with everything from soap to plant hangers), fruit and veggie stands, local animal producers, you get it…

- Your garden, your trees, gathering mushrooms and other edible plants, hunting and fishing

Well, you haven't been with me long, but I think you already know what I'm going to say:

Fast food: Never eat this crap again. Period. Break the habit. I don't care if you're starving and it's all that's open, suck it up. I don't care if the kids think it's great – this is a teaching opportunity, use it. Why? As I said earlier, it's made of the cheapest ingredients they can find – how do you think they manage to sell double cheeseburgers for a buck or less? Prisons are getting better quality food. It's filled with salt, sugar, fat and whatever else that keeps you going back. No more will be said.

Modification: There will be times of crisis and trauma in your life. Look for a Chipotle or Baja Fresh if you have no choice, but very careful.

The other three:

The supermarket – fact of life. You're going to be in there a lot, more later.

• Organic, big and little: same thing, a little more effort and usually more $$

• Gardens, etc. Yes, but…we'll talk.

Here's the deal: what you need/should/must eat for the rest of your life is just simply this: real food. Food that hasn't been processed, altered, boxed, canned or frozen, usually food that hasn't been <u>advertised</u> in any way. If you can buy it in a box, a carton, a can or a pouch, and it says "just add.." or "complete with your own…." Or "instant", or usually if it has pictures on it, don't eat it. Read the label. If any of the following show up, especially in the first few ingredients, don't buy it and don't eat it:

- high fructose corn syrup

- saturated fat

- trans fats

- partially hydrogenated oil

- sugar

- salt

- "enriched" flour

- chemicals you never heard of before

You want to eat fresh vegetables, fruit, meat, poultry, fish, bread, grains and dairy products that have been messed with as little as possible. You're going to bake it, roast it, boil it, broil it, sauté it, but never ever deep fry it. You're going to put it together and take it apart – making wonderful tasting real food, not fake chemicalized overprocessed junk that is filled with sugars, chemicals and things you can't spell or pronounce.

OK, there's going to be exceptions, I'm not the complete food Nazi. But you know what I'm talking about. (Besides, we haven't even gotten to beverages. Without chardonnay, cabernet sauvignon and tangerine juice, my life would be over. More on that later.) So let's get back to where you're going to go get all that wonderful food.

The Supermarket

Albertson's, Safeway, Wal-Mart, Kroger, Pathmark, Winn-Dixie, Publix and their colleagues make up most of them and own most of the others under different names. They have most of everything we've always shopped for – from Gold Medal flour to Calgon, and we're still going to go there. However, if you've been shopping for any time at all, you've probably noticed something. The same name market will vary enormously from neighborhood to neighborhood – some catering to an upscale clientele, some to a more working-class one, and some to an ethnic one. Some will have masa, others kimchee and others you can always find matzoh. There's a subtle difference in the quality of the produce, the types of coffee, the cuts of meat at the butcher's counter, what's in the deli and the variety of wines and beers. Some will even have the option of natural grass-fed beef, or free-range chicken in small quantities, and some won't. Try a different neighborhood next time you shop and you'll see it's true.

Remember, supermarkets and the food processing industry are partners, and they stock their shelves heavily based on what's being advertised by the different food producers and what's selling, whether it's Coke with lime, Froot Loops or Eggos. All the brands you've seen advertised on TV, in magazines, in newspapers, they're here, and almost all of them are processed and produced by the food industry, making up 80% of the food sold in supermarkets. Most of these attractively packaged and colorfully labeled products are JUNK and almost always the mixes and sauces are really easy to make with a minimum of effort, by you in the kitchen, without:

- preservatives (those things you probably can't spell and never heard of)

- chemicals(ditto)

- fillers(ditto again)

- monosodium glutamate

- emulsifiers, starches, and all those other ingredients listed on the labels that you have no earthly idea what they are

The two main reasons processed food feeds most of the country are profitability for them and convenience for you, enticed by all the advertising. You've heard those stories about Twinkies never going stale? They're true. When archeologists from 4500 A.D. excavate Denver, they could find edible Twinkies perfectly preserved, just as we did with the bog people in Ireland.

In fact, I'm 100% certain that if we took someone from 1850, princess or shopkeeper, and tried to feed them Lucky Charms or "cheese food" slices (doesn't the term "cheese food" sort of creep you out, like it's something that's supposed to be fed to small aliens that live under the basement stairs?), they'd recoil in horror and spit it out. Our taste buds and our minds have been cajoled and conditioned through advertising and repetition into believing most of the stuff for sale in supermarkets is healthy, nutritious food and nothing could be farther from the truth.

Rule of thumb in supermarkets: mostly shop the walls, not the interior aisles. The outer walls are where you will find produce, meat, and dairy. Read labels and be careful even here.

Organic Markets, Big and Little

Organic food has become a huge business in the last ten years, and will only get bigger, because we're figuring out that it's good for us, and usually tastes better, more expensive or not. As Michael Pollan talks about in "In Defense of Food", Americans spend less on food than most other people in the world. Part of that is because we're conditioned to think we shouldn't have to, but most of it is because we think, thanks to the processed and fast food industries, that we are eating well cheaply. We're NOT, and it's just that simple. Food is a huge part of your life, and makes you what you are, so be willing to spend a bit more.

If you've never been to a Whole Foods Market, or any of their upscale counterparts, you will be amazed. You feel better and healthier just stepping inside. These people have spent a lot of money to make you feel that way, and they've laid out their stores in a proven format.

First you cruise the produce aisles and see perfect, colorful vegetables and fruits that are beautifully laid out, and some maybe you've never seen before, but these people are nice, and they label them with place of origin, and you can tell your friends about Malaysian pears. The glass cases full of organic cuts of meat leave you with no guilt about eating meat, because this is meat, poultry and fish that's really had a good life before it ended up here, tenderly cared for and humanely killed.

You move on to cheeses that you never knew about, cured in small villages, perhaps in Switzerland or the Andes. Aisles and aisles of dry goods make up the middle of the store and you get a little confused here, but not to worry, because it takes a while to adapt to all the flour, pastas, cereals, spices, olives, and hundreds of brands of sauces and beans you've never heard of before, but you'll learn because you're smart and you're motivated now.

Then you get to the bakery section, and here you'll find bread that is so fragrant, delicious and crusty fresh that you throw all caution to the winds. Now this is how food should be, you'll say to yourself, loading up the cart once again. (Handy that you're near the end and that lovely bread won't get crushed, isn't it?)

Then comes the complete downfall of your wallet, because here are the deli cases. These aren't just deli cases, but restaurants. You can eat it here (there are tables and chairs for those of you who just can't wait), or take it home to heat up. There's healthy delicious entrees already prepared, salads that you wish you'd thought up, and soups –we all know how long they take to make – soups that smell so delicious you can hardly walk by them without filling up the take-out carton. This is food nirvana, and it's good for you!

Sounds like heaven, doesn't it? Except for a few things that should be obvious. First and foremost, if you shop here exclusively, you'll be spending a fortune on food, unless you're very savvy, and this takes time, trust me. You'll also be throwing some of it away be-cause: there's little preservatives in most of it, which is good, but you'll buy more than you can possibly eat in two or three days, and after that, you'll have to throw it out. So you'll learn, and after a few turns, if you're ready to change your shopping habits completely, which translates as every day or two, and only what you need, when it comes to fresh vegetables, fruits, meat and bread, you'll do all right. At first you might be spending more than you used to, (don't panic, because you will find that by not buying the processed/instant/advertised junk you may even save a few bucks, not to mention your waistline) because untainted fresh food costs a bit more, period. Why?

Because it costs more to produce it, thanks to subsidies on crops and meat, that go mostly to farms that are owned by or who sell to the big food processors. Organic farmers, whether vegetable, fruit, meat or dairy, usually spend more money to grow their crops because no matter how small their operation, they have to comply with the regulations that should really apply to the bacteria-laden huge processing farms and feedlots with all their drugs, hormones and nasty mono-culture growing and harvesting practices, even though smaller-scale farmers may care about and know more about the plants and animals they raise.

Organic farmers and ranchers can't use pesticides, drugs, hormones and chemicals, and they provide more humane conditions when it comes to raising and killing animals. (These conditions can be somewhat variable, though, and may be different from a larger farm to a smaller local one.)

However, the big food processors and the USDA are not concerned with humane conditions, from life to death; they are concerned with profits gleaned from "acceptable" guidelines. Food is simply a business, period, produced for the least amount and sold for the highest: mass production, efficiency within the legal limits of safety, cleanliness and productivity, and those legal limits are amazingly loose. Common sense will tell you if you raise a cow on a feed lot with thousands of other cows standing knee-deep in their own manure, then having to take drugs to keep them alive and healthy enough to kill because of it, instead of in a grass field the way they should be raised, that problems can ensue. All those Ecoli outbreaks make sense now, don't they?

It boils down to the common denominator, really. Safe enough, clean enough, and making a profit for the most people to feed the most people. That's the American food industry, and it isn't designed to make you healthy, it's just designed to get you fed. The food processing and advertising part of it is designed to make you feel assured about where your food comes from.

So Whole Foods and their cohorts have it right, or do they? These are the glossy organic food stores. Let's think a little further, now that we're on the good food track. What is organic food anyway? Food that's been grown or raised without pesticides, antibiotics, hormones, and isn't processed. However, you don't have to go to big organic markets to get it.

Farmer's markets are everywhere, nationwide. Fruit and veggie stands, Saturday markets and bakeries are pretty much everywhere. If you live on the coasts, fresh fish markets abound. Local livestock and dairy producers are harder to find, but they're out there too. Usually the prices are very good, better than the bigger organic stores. Do some research, on the Internet or in the newspaper. You'll be surprised, and delightfully so. Foodies are everywhere. You're about to become one.

What I've just described in the last paragraph is "little organic" – small farmers and growers, versus "big organic" – Whole Foods, Wegmans, etc. The difference may seem infinitesimal at first, but it's getting bigger every day. Wholesome food is becoming a big business, and as with all big businesses, eventually corners are cut in the name of profit, which always makes me a little nervous. I get skeptical about what somebody else's idea of quality is when it comes to profit.

Let's focus in for a moment, on a couple of the most popular and accessible of the "organic" foods. This is real food, not processed, but here's a closer look. First, bagged salad greens, most of which are sold in all supermarkets, regular and organic. This started out as iceberg lettuce with some shredded carrots (pretty much food value: zero), but has quickly moved on to some very good veggies. You can choose from radicchio, spinach, spring greens, butter lettuce, romaine, ½ and ½ mixes and even the European style mixes which make you feel oh so jetsetty.

This also started out as a very small operation delivered to local markets, sort of an off the wall packaging idea, sometime in the 1990s. It didn't stay that way long, but exploded into a huge processing industry for salad greens, and there's lots of players on the stage now with the familiar names we've heard for years, lots of our old big veggie friends. It also isn't quite as good. Ever notice no matter how far you dig through the cold case looking for the farthest date on the freshness stamp, the lettuce has brown edges or the "spring mix" greens get rather slimy in two days? I have yet to finish a bag of greens unless I've used the whole bag the first time.

Spinach was the best deal, but since the Ecoli spinach debacle, it'll take a long time for anyone to feel completely comfortable eating bagged spinach. Honestly, the whole bagged salad industry could easily have the same problems again and again. Best to go back to the produce counter or preferably, the farmers market, and buy the whole food, minus the sealed bag in which all those nasty bacteria have their own private lab to play in. If it isn't Ecoli, it could be something else, and I'd rather wash it myself anyway. Like my mother used to say, who knows where their hands have been?

My next example is the chicken and the egg. I know, that's two, but bear with me, because they're related. The poultry industry is huge, and "free range" chicken has become the watchword for getting really fresh, good-tasting and guilt-free chicken. However, at the risk of sounding like I work for PETA, I have to tell you about what the federal guidelines are for calling your chicken "free range". All this means to the more profit-oriented chicken raisers is that you have to give the chickens a small door in their cages that leads to an outside yard. Organic chickens are raised without antibiotics and growth hormones, so the chicken farmer fervently hopes his chickens don't exercise the option to check out the sky, because they could catch an infection and wipe out the whole building. Sadly, chickens aren't the most brilliant creatures, so hardly any of them ever do, they're packed in their huge stinky henhouses and don't know any better. So much for the myth of fluffy white chickens running about the pasture frolicking in the grass. If you can, find a local poultry farmer who really does let his chickens run about and eat insects and grass.

Now, the egg. We already know what the term "free range" means in the chicken business, and the other one we see a lot of lately is "cage free", which means pretty much the same thing. They're not in the usual two by two foot cages with their beaks cut off to stop them from fighting with each other (who could blame them), but put in huge sheds, tens of thousands together, but once again there's little happy clucking to be heard on the egg farm. The latest thing is "omega 3 fortified" eggs. This means they feed the chickens kelp which translates into omega 3s. If you want to pay more for any of this, go ahead, but be aware the chickens' lives are little better and you can get your omega 3 oils in lots of other ways. Again, look for a local producer.

With chickens and eggs, there's also a lot of ham – lots of the egg crates and the labels on fresh chicken have pictures of bucolic little farms with red barns under a rising sun and names like "Aunt Sallie's Homestead Farm". Cute. Call me a cynic, but sometimes the cuter the farm looks on the label the worse the conditions are.

So you see, even the best intentions sometimes backfire. The best way to insure you're eating the best and freshest food is to buy it as close to the source as you can. Sometimes (usually) this is the local produce market or farmers' markets, the big organic food store, and even your local supermarkets, some of which buy local, when they can. If it says "organic" and the price isn't astronomical, it's probably better tasting and better for you, but you're still going for the gold with fresh produce, no matter where you get it. (Except for that shiny wax on the apples – how dumb do they think we are? I suppose there's little apple gnomes that polish the suckers before they're picked? Sigh.) Just wash thoroughly, and in the case of the apple wax, scrub.

Gardens

I know what you're thinking…she's going off the deep end here. However, there's gardens and there's gardens. I've had gardens off and on for years, from Seattle to Phoenix and places in between. When things go well, they're great, and I've learned the hard way and the easy way to do them. You don't have to be a horticulturist to grow great vegetables, but it does take some work. It also turns out to be not the cheapest option – you must invest in mulch, fertilizer, seeds and plants, some tools, gloves, and a lot of time. What you do get for your time and money is the best tasting, freshest, pesticide-free vegetables you've eaten since you were a kid (or maybe ever), and a lot of personal satisfaction. So,

- You can go all the way and turn half the backyard into a flower and vegetable garden. So much for the badminton area and be ready for a LOT of work.

- Or, you can do a smaller version, anything from 8' x 4' raised boxes (Sunset Magazine has a great one, with easy to build plans, check their website), and instead of just flowers on the patio, plant veggies.

- Or, if you live in an apartment that has a patio or balcony, use pots for tomatoes and veggies, and try an herb garden. Fresh herbs taste wonderful and take little space, even a window box will do for starters.

If you decide that gardening's for you, I highly recommend a method of planting called "permaculture". This is a system that's gotten more and more popular in the last 20 years, and it basically means growing plants in harmony with each other and their environment, with things working together. Rototilling is NOT recommended or even needed to have a good garden.

For smaller gardens, you can even do a quick "instant garden". I've done these in different Western climates from mountain to desert and they've turned out very well every time. Here's the directions:

- Choose your site (sunny) and water thoroughly. Bare dirt is not necessary, you can do this right over existing weeds and grass. Cut them short, and don't use weedkillers.

- Then, spread few layers of black and white newspaper in the shape you wish to have, again, water well, but not so much that the paper falls apart. You can do rectangular beds, or circles and curves, which are pretty.

- On top of the newspaper, spread compost and mulch four to six inches deep. Be aware you're going to use lots of big bags of this stuff, and they weigh a lot, so have your friends over for a garden party, it saves your back. You can mix in a little organic fertilizer to this (chicken manure is best) and compost, but be aware that will stink for a bit, and don't overdo. Your choice.

- Plant your seeds and/or starter plants. You're done – sit back and watch things grow, keeping the soil moist with frequent watering. Not soaked, you don't have to drown things. I use soaker hoses, spread over the top of the soil, about two feet apart, but you can arrange them as you like. This method saves on water, and works very well. You can top with a thin layer of straw or grass clippings, an inch or two, to help keep the soil moist.

- You don't have to plant in "rows" as is traditional. You can make circles, figure 8s, or any pattern you want, just give each plant some room to expand.

If this sounds too good to be true, it isn't. Instant permaculture gardens are amazing. There's really no need to chop, hoe, rototill, and all that backbreaking work that we've thought had to happen for a great garden. You can use this same method for raised beds, with wood sides, if you want to get a little fancier, but the mulch will stay in place pretty well without the boxes.

Keep in mind that plants need to be thinned out (follow the seed package directions, they know what they're talking about), and that many of them need more room that you thought. Tomato plants can get big, and will need wire cages or stakes, (put them in when the plants are small), as will climbing green beans or peas. Cucumbers, zucchini and squash spread out all over the place. I haven't had good luck with root crops with this method: carrots, potatoes, beets, anything that grows below the earth – but give it a try if you really love them. Just don't expect great results.

Watering is best done with soaker hoses or by hand, because overhead sprinklers aren't good for plants, they tend to create moldy leaves and don't get to the roots. Don't overwater – your plants will look droopy if you aren't giving them enough, you'll find. Looking at your plants will tell you everything you need to know.

The very best thing of all with instant gardens is: very few weeds!

Fruit trees are quite possibly the best thing on earth. From apples to oranges, there's nothing like them. Depending on your climate, pears, apples, peaches, cherries, oranges, lemons, grapefruit, limes and tangerines are there for the picking. If you don't grow them in your yard, there's lots of people that do, and lots of orchards that have you-pick times, all across the country. In the southwest, citrus trees are part of the landscaping in most green belts and subdivisions, and you can take a walk and pick a bagful in a few minutes, and no one minds. I grew up in the Midwest, and my neighbors always wanted someone to pick their apples so they didn't have to clean them up later.

Strawberry and raspberry fields often have you-pick days, and love to have people come and pluck the little darlings. For a minimal amount of work, you can have fresh berries by the pailful for little money, instead of paying up to $5 for a 6 ounce plastic box of them.

If you want to find out more about gardening and particularly permaculture, bookstores have lots of garden books, and the Internet has great permaculture sites to explore. Start with www.permaculture.net. Permaculture has changed lives around the world, from Australia to Africa, helping people grow enough food to eat in some cases for the first time in their lives.

Hunting and Gathering

I grew up in Michigan, the heartland of deer hunting, so I know how this works. Every fall, perfectly sane men, (and some women) go nuts – they head for the deer camp cabin. I'm not sure what goes on at the deer camp but I think there's a lot of "male bonding", poker, beer, and farting along with the hunting. Sometimes they bring home venison and expect their wives and girlfriends to produce fabulous meals out of it, and sometimes this happens. Years of learning about salt water soaks and lots of cookbooks go into this magic trick, and some pretty good dinners are produced.

From the standpoint of fresh and un-messed with food, hunting – whether it's deer, elk, bear or road kill of indeterminate varieties, is unparalleled. Whether you want to eat it or not is the question.

Most of us, particularly those of us who have opted to live in larger cities, don't relish the taste of the wild. It's a little different than beef, pork or chicken, and we aren't used to it. There's been a surge in restaurants lately that offer wild game at big prices, and they seem to be doing well, but cooking it at home hasn't really followed. If you like it, it's lean and free of any of the antibiotics and hormones that the commercial meat industry allows, so go for it.

I grew up with a father who was a big game hunter, and deer was the tip of the iceberg for this man. Bear, bighorn sheep and elk were his hunting challenge and he was good at it. I learned to shoot a rifle at the tender age of ten (he'd grown weary of not having a son and opted for me), but his idea of deer camp was a ten room hunting lodge that usually housed corporate clients, albeit the bearskin rugs and antlered heads on the walls. It wasn't for me, and he grudgingly but kindly acquiesced.

However, years later when I moved west, I became close friends with a couple who hunted, but this was a different sort of hunting altogether. They were both professional people who did this every year. He would go up a week early, into the River of No Return Wilderness Area, in a four wheel drive pulling a trailer with two of their horses, and set up camp – a large tent with a double featherbed cot, a case of French wine, many candles, and a well-stocked kitchen, replete with herbs and copper pans, among other amenities. She would arrive, and together they would hunt deer and elk, using only bows and arrows. This respite from civilization invigorated them, and they came back not only renewed but with a freezer full of food which they knew how to cook, and the dinners I enjoyed at their home were incredible.

Mushrooms are the other favorite of wild food gatherers. I love mushrooms, but I don't know a thing about good ones from ones that will drop you in your tracks, so I don't do this. If you decide to hunt wild mushrooms, find knowledgeable experts in this field, and learn from them. Wild mushrooms are wonderful – they taste like nothing else, with a tang of earth and something solely their own, but knowing what you're doing when finding them is absolutely essential.

Whenever I see plump juicy blackberries for sale in the grocery store, I think back to all the blackberry bushes growing by the side of the road when I was kid. We used to pick them on the way home from school. You can still find them all over the country, in parks (Seattle is great for this, and so is northern California), in overgrown backyards and along country roads. Grab a basket or a pail, and go out and pick some, they're wonderful. You can put them in salads, a pie, or make some jam. You'll be glad you did.

Here's the thing – keep your eyes open. Great food grows wild everywhere, you just have to recognize it, and pick it. I remember my high school biology teacher bringing puffballs to class, which we cut up and cooked with butter and garlic and right then I decided I loved mushrooms. Sometimes it takes knocking on a door and asking permission, which is usually gratefully granted (most people can never use all the produce on their landscaping and want somebody to take it away, especially for free), or some negotiation may be

required. Tell them you're working on a biology proj-
ect, or better yet, writing a book.

□□□□

Whew. We're done talking about food, right and
wrong, (until Chapter 7). I know, this was a lot to digest (no pun intended). I'm going to have a list of web-
sites and books at the end. (No fair flipping there now
and leaving my pearls of wisdom to hang out because
we're not done yet.) Food is no minor matter – it's our
fuel, our lifesource, and sometimes, our passion.

We spend more time gathering it, whether from
Safeway, Kroger, Farmer Joe, or our backyards – then
cooking it, and the joy of eating it, whether at home or
over at La Trattoria, then anything else we do. Oh yes
– you think every Wednesday the local paper devotes
an entire section to "Food" because they just feel like
it? Or the Restaurant Review isn't the most-read section in any paper or magazine? Or that Martha Stewart's Living and every other magazine at the checkout
that has a cover filled with luscious recipes is there by
accident? We live in a contradictory world – eat and

be thin. That's just one of the reasons why I said the cards are stacked against you. Once you understand that, you're ready.

Let's start doing it smart. It'll be a joy, which is what it's meant to be. This huge part of your life should never be a guilt-ridden, calorie-counting food exchange trial. With food, we're going where it should always be:

- Good for you
- Tasting fantastic
- Helping you feel great, physically and mentally
- Making you look great

Genetically Modified Foods

No book about food and diet would be complete without talking about this. It's a pretty big controversy, and one I can't fail to address. One of the reasons I promote organic food, big and little, over everyday supermarkets, is this very subject.

The majority of corn, cottonseed oil, canola, and soy grown in the United States is now genetically engineered and modified. Corn in particular finds its way into most of the processed food in this country, from starch, flour, cereal to corn syrup, which by the way is the sweetener in most sodas, baked goods, processed food dinners and even cereals. If you shop exclusively at major supermarkets, you will be eating genetically modified food, no question. Organic markets aren't exclusively immune from this either, but they try to be.

As of yet, most of the fresh vegetables and fruits available are not part of this equation, but as time passes, I have no doubt they will be, and so far there is no labeling or notification required for the consumer.

Whether this is a problem for your health is yet to be determined, scientifically. There's a lot of arguing going on, pro and con. As far as I'm concerned, however, whenever there's this much debate, that's a good reason to not eat anything that you know is GM food.

I'm sure the food producers and the federal government are looking out for our best interests on this, but I also have Rumpelstiltskin locked in the study spinning gold from straw. When it comes to profits, people do funny things.

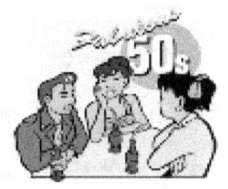

Soda Pop Sluts
A Faerie Tale

Once upon a time, in the land of USA, the farmers were happy and productive. They were so productive, especially with the golden ears of corn they grew, that soon they surpassed even the king's wildest dreams of how much corn they could possibly grow. All the greatest wizards in the land put their heads together to figure out what was to be done with all that huge surplus of corn. Mounds of the stuff were molding away all over the land and it was expensive to ship, not to mention smelling bad.

Well, it didn't take too long. Corn can be made into syrup, specifically "high fructose corn syrup". The wizards then discovered HFCS, as they lovingly called it for short, can be put into almost anything that people eat, in place of sugar and more cheaply, too. It's especially wonderful for sodas, which the people loved.

Another group of wizards was involved in making food fast, packaged, processed and convenient. At first, they started with simple stuff, but once they discovered HFCS, they put it just about everything they made, and discovered the people loved it just as much as the sodas they drank when they ate it.

There were a couple of wizards who kept droning on about nutrition and obesity and a responsibility towards the health of the people, but they were quietly and efficiently turned out of the kingdom by the court jesters who made advertisements. Nobody wants to listen to boring statistics when they're eating cheeseburgers, French fries, and sugar-coated cereals, not to mention the great taste of Coke and Pepsi.

The king and his advisors gave lots of money to the farmers to keep growing way too much corn,(called subsidies) so the food processors could make HFCS and put it in lots and lots of foods, and those royal edicts continue to this very day.

So, in the land of USA even today, some thirty years later or so, a few people are richer, and everyone is happy, and…..much fatter, spending more time going to doctors and worrying about their cholesterol and blood pressure.

(Television and video games helped a lot with that, too, cause it's really fun to sit on your ass, eat chips and dips and wash it down with gallons of HFCS sweetened soda. Hello worried populace on diets, goodbye playing outside.)

Chapter 5
You Don't Get Any Pudding

We're getting down to it now, but don't be scared. You know what you're supposed to eat, you know why, and you know where to get it. Now it's the hard part. Just because you can, doesn't mean you should. Isn't that the hardest part of just about everything in life? How much you eat is a major factor in what you weigh, how you feel, and how you look. But, it's not as hard as you think, and I'm going to give you some information and tools to make it a lot easier, and practically painless. Think French, or just about any other place but right here in the good old USA, land of excess and fat people.

We've been brainwashed since childhood and it's still a constant bombardment. Three meals a day, the food groups, the USDA food pyramids, Madison Avenue and its advertising – from Good Housekeeping magazine to McDonald's:

- Eat and you'll feel better.

- Finish your plate and make Mom happy, children in China are starving

- I missed lunch, and I'm starving, so I can eat a big dinner.

- If you don't eat breakfast, you'll never lose weight.

- Always eat well balanced nutritional meals, including dessert.

- Let's celebrate – hey, it's a holiday, which means lots of whatever you want.

- Snacks are your right and you should have them to keep your energy up.

- Eat – it's GOOD for you.

No, it's not. Not necessarily, and certainly not with those guidelines, threats, coercions and admonitions. There's reasons we live in the fattest country in the history of the world, and a few of them are listed above. Let's take a look at the size of your stomach, shall we?

It's not all that big, for starters. Average size 6" long x 12" around. About a quart. But it has an amazing capacity to expand. A good guideline is to make a fist. No matter what size you are, Shaquille or America's Next Top Model – your fist is about the size of your stomach, more or less. It's going to grow as you fill it, but that's where the trick comes in – not only what you fill it with, but how much. You know how dogs will eat until there's nothing left in the bowl? Well, people have pretty much the same problem. The trick is to not fill the bowl. Here's some guidelines:

- 3 oz. of meat, average portion, is about the size of a pack of cigarettes.

- 1 cup of potatoes, pasta, rice, a tortilla, or a slice of bread is about the size of a baseball.

- Vegetables and fruit you can gauge for yourself but remember there's a lot of water in most vegetables that doesn't count, especially lettuces.

As you can see, if you ate a 3 oz. filet mignon, a small baked potato and a small green salad with say, balsamic vinaigrette, you just filled your stomach, and might even squeeze in a tiny slice of cheesecake. Not so bad. On the other hand, if you opted for a T-bone at 10 oz., potatoes au gratin, three slices of garlic bread, and corn on the cob along with a salad globbed with blue cheese or ranch dressing, and then a piece of apple pie with ice cream, you were the dog with the big bowl. Your stomach is now at least twice the size it was before you sat down, and you don't just feel satisfied, you feel stuffed. That's because you are, and it's not pretty.

There's an infinite number of variations on this theme, but the latter one above is the average American dinner. The same holds true for breakfast and lunch. For example, a hearty American breakfast is two eggs, three slices of bacon, hash browns, two slices of toast, and a stack of pancakes. Or, lunch is a sandwich that is piled with sliced meat, cheese, tomatoes and lettuce with a side of potato chips and/or potato salad, a piece of fruit and maybe a cookie or two? Maybe every single thing on the menu is fresh, organic and prepared well, but there's simply too much of it.

We've been conditioned to think this is abundant, healthy, all-American eating. It's what restaurants sell us, and what we've been conditioned to think of as a complete meal, and if it's less, we feel cheated.

Unless you're a lumberjack, an athlete, a ditchdigger, or doing some sort of heavy labor for the day, you don't need to eat anywhere near this much food. But amazingly enough, we do, because we're programmed to think we're supposed to. You're going to feel sluggish, uncomfortable, take antacids and fall asleep at your desk around 3 o'clock and in front of the TV around 8:30.

Here's what you do instead: you want a hearty breakfast, try one egg, one slice of bacon, one piece of toast, and a piece of fruit. On other days, try oatmeal or another good cereal (read the labels) and a piece of fruit, or yogurt. For lunch, have half a sandwich along with a cup of soup or a small green salad. We already covered the dinner option. You aren't going to starve, get malnutrition, or freak out and eat a whole carton of Hagen-Daz. You are, however, going to be alert, not have gas and bloating, or trouble with your waistband mysteriously shrinking during the day. Your stomach will thank you, and so will every other organ in your body that doesn't have to work overtime.

Think of it this way: never eat more than three baseballs at any meal. Two is much better, and remember the size of your fist.

▢▢▢▢

Restaurants are wonderful, and I love them, not just because the food is great, service is nice, but because I get great ideas for stuff to cook at home. (Sometimes, I love to take a small notebook with me and not very surreptitiously scribble in it after I've tried something. Word spreads quickly through the restaurant that you could be a food critic and occasionally the service improves. Try this, it's fun.)

The only problem is restaurant portions are, for the most part, huge – much more food is given you than any normal person should eat. Italian restaurants are the best at this – the average pasta portion could feed a family of three and on top of that, there's most likely antipasto, salad, and garlic bread, to say nothing of tiramisu. Your stomach, and I don't care who you are, should never expand this much. You wonder why all those guys on The Sopranos are the size of Sumo wrestlers and complaining of heartburn all the time? Carmela might cook it, but she sure doesn't eat much of it, and that's who you want to emulate, not Tony.

So what should you do? There are a lot of great restaurants that have figured this out, and serve portions and great food according. There's many more that haven't. So, when you go to a restaurant, unless it's the nouvelle cuisine sort, or one that's got some idea of quality rather quantity, only eat half the portion you're served. Ask for a takeout container for the rest, if it's worth it. Or, if you're with a friend who knows better, as you do, split the entrée. This is becoming more and more common, so don't be intimidated. Waiters are used to it, and don't mind bringing a second plate. Besides, you're saving the price of a second entrée, and you can overtip a bit, so if you do get attitude, don't go back. New restaurants open every day, while others close.

Avoid buffets, or if you can't, be careful because these are dangerous. If you end up at one, and you find yourself losing control, try getting just a little bit of the most appealing items. Or, sometimes what looked great on the serving table tastes awful when you get back to your seat, so take one bite and pass. It's not like you ordered the entrée, and the buffet people are used to this, so don't worry about offending anyone. After all, it is about choices, and they should always be yours, not anybody else's.

We're conditioned to think in terms of certain amounts of food, a full plate, for example. Well, plate sizes vary wildly and there's been a wave in home décor lately to make even bigger dinner plates. This is wonderful, if you want to artfully arrange the food, and drizzle sauces in patterns on the plate. This is awful if you just fill it up with big portions. The weird thing is, people tend to eat what's on the plate. It's conditioning. Remember the dog bowl?

If you aren't going to be artful, or you're one of those people like my sister who freaks if any food touches any other food on her plate, use the salad plate instead. I'm serious as a heart attack about this. Excuse the pun, but remember it.

The last thing to remember is timing. Most of us eat like jailhouse cons. For some reason I can't fathom, unless we're in a restaurant or at a dinner party, where there's lots of conversation, we shovel it in like somebody's going to swipe it if we don't fork it first. Slow down. I know, probably everybody from your mom to the last diet book you read says the same thing, but on this they're right. The fact is this: your stomach doesn't tell your brain that it's full for twenty minutes after you ate the food. Believe this, it's true, and I'm not saying it again. When you go for that third slice of pizza, it's probably because you wolfed down the first two, and what the hell, it's there just looking at you, saying "Eat me." Get over it, Alice. Wait 17 minutes. You'll find you don't really want or need any more to eat. The pizza's not going anywhere. You are.

You're going to eat less. To recap, here's exactly how you're going to do it:

- Nobody will starve anywhere if you don't clean your plate. Remember: you don't need it, you've just been programmed to think you do. Walk away.

- Ignore all food advertising, no matter where you see it.

- Just because it's "time" – lunch or dinner, doesn't mean you have to eat if you're not really hungry.

- Cut your portions in half.

- Use restaurants for great food, fun and research, not stuffing yourself – split the meal, leave it or take home a doggie bag.

- Use smaller plates or get artful with decorative touches.

- Sloooow down.

- If you can't resist the lobster bisque or foie gras, just take one or two bites, then you've had that wonderful food and you're done.

- Most importantly, eat only the food you really want to eat, so you don't feel cheated, but remember the baseballs.

Once you start doing this, you're going to get up from the table, and want to take a walk with your dog, your kids, your significant other, not sit down on the couch and collapse. You can go outside and play with the kids instead of sitting on the patio and watching them; you're going to feel good physically, and that translates into feeling good mentally. Good all around. Remember: great food doesn't have to be eaten in large quantities to be enjoyed. It'll come around again soon.

Chapter Six

Dancing with Wolves:
Learning to Move Your Ass
and Growing to Love it

Yes, it's the exercise part, but don't put the book-mark in and leave me here. I've told you the truth so far, haven't I?

Maybe you've been looking forward to this..... maybe not. You probably think there's going to be lots of pictures and diagrams, talk of gym equipment and weights, treadmills, benchpresses, spandex and en-couragement to try out for the Boston Marathon after you've gotten used to running at least three miles ev-ery morning.

I can't frankly think of anything worse. No offense to those who've been training for any marathon, however there's many many ways to exercise that are enjoyable, fun, and practical that don't involve getting up at 4 or 5 AM and running in nasty weather, bad neighborhoods, dealing with dogs that people let out to crap in other people's yards before anyone's awake, and pleading with your neighbor to go with you so you're not lonely or scared. I used to do this, and it was hell. Also it lasted about two weeks every time.

Here's the thing. You must do something physically active at least five days out of seven every week for at least 30 minutes that gets your heart rate up, gets your blood flowing, and gets your muscles warm and loosened up to be in good physical condition and lose weight. (I'd frankly recommend six out of seven for an hour, but let's start with something you can live with and you'll move up to that.) This does not mean scrubbing the kitchen floor or getting in a fight with your husband/boyfriend/the possums in your backyard. You can march in place to John Philip Sousa and the Marine Band for 30 minutes if that's what you're into, but there are more interesting options.

The Gym

I know what you're thinking: it's too expensive, it's a meat market, there's all these thin women wearing pink spandex, I'll have cameltoe in these pants and feel out of place and people will think I'm a geek. Wrong. Here's how it really is:

There's a plethora of gyms operating nationally – LA Fitness, 24 Hour Fitness, Gold's, Prime Time Fitness, and Curves (which is just women) and many others that have figured out their client base is everyone, not just hotties looking to hook up. I've been to most of them, and I've been pleasantly surprised. Nobody cares how you look or what shape you're in. There's everyone from 80-year-olds doing ten pound squats to Mr. America hopefuls lifting 200 pounds. Most of these outfits have pools, saunas and babysitting, and usually it's free with membership, which is amazingly cheap, from $20-25 a month, there's lots of "sales" with no signup fee and you can go as often as you want. (I think most of the gym people work on commission, and negotiating is good. Remember, you don't ask, you don't get.) Also, they usually offer a free personal trainer analysis, with some guy that looks like Taye Diggs or Daniel Craig, which is pretty painless, to get started with, so you can figure out how the machines work and what you need to do, and there's free classes, which range from hip-hop to yoga to water aerobics.

The downside of this wonderfulness is that gyms are usually crowded from 5-8 AM in the morning, and very crowded from 5-8 PM at night, which is when most people stop in after work. The real downside is that you may not get in the car and actually go, which is the real deal-breaker with gyms. (If you carry a bag in the car, with a pair of sweat pants, t-shirt and shoes, it will help.)

If you join, and if you actually go, after a couple of weeks it'll be a habit you won't want to give up. From the machines, which are incredible, to the classes, which are fun, you'll find you get really comfortable with the place, the people, and the whole setup. You'll be a regular, sort of like Cheers without the alcohol and the know-it-all fat guy. You'll start to share experiences – like sore muscles turning into visible ones, who hogs the benchpress, and whether the pool water is too warm. The real plus is you're going to start to see your body changing.

You will have shoulder definition, which is really sexy, your underarms will stop sagging, your thighs will be getting defined and hard, and your waistline will shrink as your breasts rise. The real pluses are things you can't see – a change in your heart rate, better cholesterol rate, more lung capacity, and a general attitude change. Yeah, those machines work

Maybe you're lucky enough to have a gym where you work, some people do, and it's free. My experience with gyms started out at the University of Washington Huskies training center on my lunch hour. It was great, football players are seriously in shape and a lot of fun, and many of them were very helpful, and full of good advice. (Tip: never use those leg-lifting machines with bars, they're very hard on the knees.)

But, if you get bored, can't go on your lunch hour or later, or don't want to pay at least $25 a month or so, here's the next option, especially since you already know what you need to do, and which muscles you need to work.

The Gym – Option Two

You don't live in a city or a town where they have gyms. You live in a small town, a village, the woods, the country, on a farm, the beach, Mexico – all good places, but not ones that cater to people working out. Or, you just don't like going out to exercise with other people around, or you can't get there easily. So, make your own.

Home gyms, and I use the term really loosely, are simple, inexpensive and easy to set up.

- First, you need a space (your bedroom will do, or the spare room, living room, family room, den, patio or basement), big enough where you can move around a little, spread out your arms, take a few paces left, right, back and forth, without knocking over a lamp or crashing into a wall – basically a <u>minimum</u> of a six foot circle.

- Then, you need some free weights – I use five pounders, but you can start with three. Also ankle weights, usually five pounds, for leg work.

- A rubber mat – yoga ones are best, they have good cushion and traction. You can

get them at most discount stores like Mar-
shall's for $10.

- A DVD player and TV, if you want to use
  DVDs, which I highly recommend over
  learning exercises from a book, even this
  one.

- Wear whatever you're comfortable in – I
  love cotton, because it breathes, and I usually wear a tank top and shorts, or sweat-
  pants, depending on the season. Fashion
  statements they are not and on early morn-
  ings, even jammies work fine.

That's the basics. If you have room, even in a different area, get a stationary exercise bike, treadmill,
elliptical machine, or Nordictrack. Don't groan and
think you're going to spend a fortune. I got my bike
from Goodwill for $10 and it's great. I've never gone
to a thrift store that didn't have lots of exercise equipment for practically nothing. Sadly, people invest a lot
of money in this stuff, never use it, and give it to thrift
stores. (The choices are especially good in the spring,
when people start getting tired of seeing that stuff they
got for Christmas gathering dust, or realize their New
Year's resolutions are deader than two week old pink-
dyed Easter chicks.) More expensive exercise equip-

ment moves through America's thrift stores every day for pennies than is sold at retail for hundreds of dollars, guaranteed.

Now, what to do. What follows is a good basic workout using lighter weights and a combination of exercises that I have found works very well, and all it costs you is your time and some sweat. After three weeks of doing this every other day, you're going to find you've got sexy shoulder definition, better looking arms, a flatter stomach, and harder thighs. Don't stop – it only gets better from there.

I'm going to explain this assuming that you've never seen a workout DVD, been to a gym, or just want to start at the beginning, Alice. If you have some experience, then this is going to be much clearer for you, and if you don't understand what I'm saying, get a DVD or two, check the Internet for exercises, or stop in at the gym and observe. You'll catch on fast, because this isn't rocket science, trust me – everybody at a gym would like to make you think differently, because they make money doing so, but it's plain truth and common sense.

Warm-up

Yes, really. This works, and helps you not have sore muscles the next day. When you start using muscles, they produce lactic acid as a self-defense, and to help dispense this you need to warm up and cool down afterwards. So, stand up, put your feet about 2' apart, and swing your arms around in a circle like you're flying, first frontwards, then backwards. Do this about ten times each, big circles. Then, stretch your arms out over your head straight up and down, ten times. Now, bend at the waist and put your right hand on your left ankle. Count to five. Straighten up, then reach down again, with your left hand on your right ankle. Do this ten times each. As you get more stretched out, put your palms on the floor beside each foot. (It will happen.) Then, straighten up, feet shoulder width apart, arms hanging normally, and breathe. Bend over from the waist, let your arms dangle and stay there for a few seconds. Stand up straight. You're ready. (In all of this, keep your knee joints loose, never locked. Don't worry if you can't reach your ankles the first few times, go as far as you can, and it'll get better as you go.)

Arms, Shoulders

Using hand weights, pick up one in each hand, and don't overgrip. Standing straight, arms at your sides, palms down, lift your arms together to shoulder height out in front of you, arms straight. Hold for a second or two and then bring your arms down. Repeat 12 times. Do this slowly, to a count of eight, four up and four down.

Standing straight, arms at your sides, palms down, lift your arms straight out to the sides, shoulder height. Use the same count. Repeat 12 times. I have a friend who combines these two moves: Bring arms out from sides, move to the front (touch the weights together), move back to each side, then down.

For that underarm flabby stuff, here's the one: Put one foot up on a two foot high chair, couch, whatever. Bend over slightly. Pick up weight in the opposite hand, pull elbow up, then turn weight so your palm is up, and stretch your arm behind you and up as high as you can. Hold for a second, (to make this extra effective, pulse your elbow up and down a few times).

Return to start and repeat 12 times on each side. Again, same eight count. This really works.

These are the big three exercises and will get your arms in shape in no time. For more definition, sculpting, all that wonderful stuff, keep going, and investigate others. I say do 12 times each, but that's just the beginning. Weight people say 12 times is a "set", so do three sets of each of these after a while and you'll really take off. When it gets too easy, use heavier weights. Rest for one minute between sets, this lets the muscles replenish. You will NOT get muscle-bound or look like you've been taking steroids. You will look good. (If you do want to get really muscled, use heavier weights and/or start doing bench presses at the gym. I prefer the lean, dancer look, but each to his own.)

Stomach, Abs

Stomach exercises are not fun. No way, no how. But they do work, and there's a great satisfaction in that. There's a lot of different ones, but I like these. Pilates core exercises are very effective, and these are variations of that. Here's three:

Leg lift: Lie down on your back, with a mat. Lift your legs up all the way, at right angle to the rest of you. Stretch your arms down towards your butt, palms up, lift your head and shoulders, and pulse, moving your arms towards where your feet would have been. Keep your lower back flat on the mat. Do 100 of these. Take your time, do it in groups of 25. They aren't hard. Start with 50 if they're killing you.

Bicycle: Lie down on your back. Keeping your back flat, lift your legs, bending your knees. Put arms behind your head, hands clasped. Lift up head and shoulders, and move your legs as though you were riding a bike, touching left elbow to right knee, and vice versa. Do 25 on each side.

Crunch and variation: Lie down on your back, knees bent and lifted, keeping back flat on floor. Put your arms behind your head, hands clasped. Using stomach muscles, lift your head and shoulders towards your knees. Go as far as you can. Do 25. Then, lean both your legs to right side, touching floor. Lift your head and shoulders towards opposite side from knees, as though your elbows were trying to touch the floor. (Don't worry, they never will.) Do 25. Do the same on the other side.

Legs

Lie on your side, legs extended, head propped on elbow, your other arm in front of you at your waist. Balance yourself, don't lean too far forward. Bend lower leg at a right angle at the knee, and keeping your upper leg straight, raise as high as you can, foot flexed. Do 30 of these. Then, put upper leg towards front about a foot, and pulse up and down (about three inches) 30 times. Then, do the same with the upper leg, behind you about a foot. Do the same on the other side.

When you feel ready, try this for an extra challenge: Put both legs together, and lift them off the floor as high as you can, raising your upper body at the same time, in a jackknife type position. Do as many as you can. Works legs and abs, fabulous.

Cool Down

Stand straight, and position yourself like an "x", with arms and legs extended. Moving slowly, wave your arms around you as though you held a veil, flowing from side to side, bending your knees at the same time. After a time, bend over at the waist and let your arms dangle, breathing slowly. Stretch up to the sky, feeling your blood tingle through your arms and legs. Shake out your arms and legs, breathing evenly. You just did something wonderful for yourself.

If you've never exercised before, start with fewer reps of each exercise I've described here, and build up to more. I'm not wearing black leather and standing over you with a whip, for Pete's sake. Don't do anything that hurts, or feels like you've gone too far or done too much. Common sense is your guide, use it. Your heart rate should go up, and you should sweat by the time you're done. You're going to be a little sore in the next day or two, but don't let that stop you. No, you didn't "pull" anything, have kidney disease or hurt yourself, you're just sore from using muscles that you haven't used in a while, maybe ever. They'll adjust, and the more you use them, they better they'll feel. It's true, even if when you say to yourself, "Oh I can't exercise today, my muscles are just hurting too much." Bull. Keep it going and don't be a complete pussy. Think Sparta, not Athens.

Do these exercises <u>every other day,</u> not daily. The muscles need to rest. On the other days, do something aerobic, which means move your ass. Suggestions follow.

Yoga

Yoga is best way in the world to become flexible, get long lean muscles, better breathing capacity, ease aches and pains (especially your back), lower your blood pressure, de-stress, be energized, relaxed, and all around in the best physical condition you can be. For a long time I kept hearing this from my friends, doctors, and physical therapists, but for some unknown reason, I resisted. Lots of people do, because: it looks difficult, it looks boring, it's sort of odd, it originated in a different culture, and if you go to a yoga class people will think you're stupid and/or clumsy. Well, none of this is true, except that it originated in India, and yoga has a long long history because it WORKS.

You can learn yoga from a DVD. To get really excited about it, though, the best way to learn yoga is at a yoga studio. They all offer beginning classes, or a three week introduction to yoga, which not only teach you the basic poses, but the good ones also tell you the history of this amazing form of exercise, why it's good for you, and exactly how to do it, and what it can do for you, which is very valuable.

So, spend the money, it's minimal, and learn the basics. You'll have this knowledge for a lifetime. You can continue to go to the studio, classes are usually an hour and around $10-12. Or, you can do it at home as well – all you need is a mat and the small space I described earlier. Any accoutrements, like music, lighting, sound and scent, you can add as you go. I sometimes use candles, incense, a small water fountain, and chakra meditation music, something from Krishna Das or Carolyn Myss,(check Amazon.com) but you can start with none of these things and add them as you like, or not.

You need to wear clothing you can move in, cotton or cotton mix pants that are comfortable and not binding, and a t-shirt or cami that doesn't constrict your upper body. That's it – yoga is always done barefoot.

If you're still skeptical, let me tell you about my first intro to yoga class. I was pretty apprehensive, and showed up to find ten other people who pretty much felt the same way. There were four men, and seven women, in all shapes, sizes and ages, from 20 to 60, and relatively thin to heavyweight. Trust me, these didn't look like people who had worked out, ever. The room was pleasantly warm, with a wooden floor, dim lighting and very clean. We all grabbed mats and blankets from the cupboards and made our spaces, as directed, and within two hours were the happiest eleven people on the planet, relaxed, laughing, secure and couldn't wait to come back the next week, wishing it were the next day.

Yeah, we were all a little sore the next day or two, as we were told we would be, because we were stretching and using muscles that we never knew we had. But, I still see at least seven of those people now and then when I go to the yoga studio, and we all know we were given a wonderful gift.

I have no doubt that if every person in America did a yoga practice for an hour even three times a week, the number of visits to doctors and psychologists, traffic accidents, (especially during commuting time), divorces, assaults, child abuse, teenage trauma, and damn near every other damaging thing that people do to each other and themselves would be cut in half if not more. I'm not kidding. Try it and you'll see. OK, unless you're a psychopath, (not sure it would've helped Ted Bundy), but there's always a contingency factor in everything.

Dance

Think back to when you were a child. You danced all the time, whether it was to your parents' Bill Haley, Led Zeppelin, Duran Duran, swing music or jazz. You had the best time, you flung your arms out, you twirled, you stomped, you grooved, and you loved it. You still would, but perhaps you forgot. Or maybe, when you got to be a teenager, self-consciousness took over, and you started worrying about what people thought about your efforts and your dance moves, which were supposed to take on a certain style or shape, and maybe you quit dancing altogether, unless it was somebody's wedding or you were behind three martinis.

But, even now, when you're in a store or in the car and some song comes on the radio, you start to move your hips and shoulders. Your body didn't forget, and it wants to move. Dance, no matter what form it takes, is instinctual in the human mind and body. Most societies that aren't so focused on doing the socially or politically correct thing or making a buck still dance like crazy. They know it makes people happy. Quit repressing it, and get back to it. You don't have to do it for anybody but yourself, (at least until you get really good at it). Here's some ways to get down to it:

- Turn on the radio, or put on a CD, and start moving. If you're out of practice, do it when no one's around, but do it. Go for at least 20 minutes, and really get into it. Wiggle, jump, shake those hips and shoulders. Nobody cares what you look like or how you move. Just work up a sweat. If you're concerned at all about style and want to take your show on the road to the club, start watching MTV and movies, and copy them. It's easier than it looks. If you want heavy beats and drums, try anything by Gabrielle Roth. (My personal favorite is "Tribe".) This is amazing stuff. She uses it in her studio to get people moving and in touch with themselves and is impossible to not move your body when you hear it.

- Take dance classes. Dancing with the Stars and all the other TV shows are extremely popular, and people are enjoying learning or re-learning how to dance. Once you've started moving, you might want some more advanced ways to do it. There's ballet, salsa, hip-hop, tango, African dance, tap, ballroom, hula, swing, jazz, so many others. You do NOT need a partner. Just sign up and go. I was apprehensive about this too, but once I got there, it was fine. Many of these dance styles are really disguised exercise classes. For the others, most people didn't have partners, they were just like me and simply wanted to learn a dance style. Teachers and studios are used to singles, and the classes are geared to this. My first salsa class we traded partners every ten minutes, and I still go to salsa clubs to dance and find my old partners from class now and then. Swing dance clubs usually have a lesson the first thing every night as well, and you get a partner that usually doesn't know any more than you do. You'll find you're having a great time and learning as you go. People who have learned to shed their inhibitions and dance want to keep doing it, and they're extremely supportive of each other. It's just fun and that's all that matters.

• Belly dance – whether it's Turkish, Arabian, Egyptian, American Tribal, or tribal fusion, there's many variations – it's the most fun, sensual, waistline trimming, body firming, make you feel good about yourself type of dance there is. Bare that belly, love it, and regain your soul. You don't need any fancy clothes to start – the usual tank top and pants, and if you want to jingle when you move your hips, an inexpensive belt with coins and bling. (Later on, you can go nuts with amazing costumes and finger cymbals (zills) if you want). This dance in some form is the oldest in the world and there's a reason why. Its pure sensuality makes women feel good about themselves, sexy, fluid and free, and makes men dream, awakening something instinctual in everyone that does it as well as those who watch it performed. Belly dance has been done everywhere from Grecian caves to desert campfires to modern American stages, and the delight it evokes it always the same. This is NOT stripping, or exotic dancing, or something shameful. This IS joyous, beautiful, sensual, freeing and a dance that takes skill and dedication to learn, but the learning is an experience you'll look forward to every class. The added benefit is that when people find out you're a belly dancer, women can't wait to ask you about it and where you dance, and men look at you with new eyes. Trust me on this. (It can also lead to sun tattoos around your navel.)

- Just get out and dance – go with your girlfriends, a group of friends from work, or
your boyfriend/husband (get his ass moving, too, he'll love it) – country line, rock,
swing, hip-hop or salsa, clubs are everywhere. Have a good time.

There's so many more ways to exercise, and here's
few I've tried and liked, and some I've watched others
do and winced, but exercise and sports are extremely
individualistic, and one person's fun and dedication is
another's worst nightmare:

- Karate. You're going to work hard, get
sweaty, and eventually get fit. You're probably not going to be kicking ass like Buffy
the vampire slayer, but the thought's there.
Most karate studios get you on a track toward being a black belt (ooooh) but they
emphasize that this is a "defensive" system
because nobody wants to get sued for turning out assassins or vigilantes, so you're not
going to be too dangerous unless you really
work it. The black belt test I went to had
people moving like they were in slow-mo
(which isn't going to scare off any muggers)
getting the moves right, and when the test-
ees couldn't break the boards, they let them

do it over and over until they finally broke a couple and called it good. Let's face it, the grading system from belt to belt is designed to make money for the karate studio, because it keeps you paying for classes, buying the stuff, and doing the certifications as you progress. This is fine, I guess, if you really like it, but don't be fooled into thinking it's anything else. This is a business like lots of others. There's exceptions to the rule, like always, but the grand master from Karate Kid is hard to find. Wax on, wax off. Do some research on who's teaching you.

- Tai Chi. This is pretty nifty stuff. It's an old Asian exercise system that is based on fluid movements, and you've probably seen it in movies before, even if you didn't know what it was. Good old David Carradine from Kung Fu fame (grasshopper, take the pebble from my hand) has DVDs and there's a lot of classes available. It 's easy to get started, and tends to be something that people continue to do, because they like it, it works, and it's pretty much free, once you learn the basics, sort of like yoga. When I lived in Seattle, there was a group of people who did it every Sunday morning under the Interstate 5 freeway overpasses in the University District (it's usually raining, so that was a good place), and I hear they still do. People would come by and just join in,

and everybody had a great time – it's wonderful exercise, relaxing, and subtly very
good at gaining muscle, balance, and breath
control. I know dancers and actors who
do it every day. In China, there's classes
in many cities every morning as the sun
comes up in the town squares, and people
just come. Nighttime, too.

- Fencing. It's been around for centuries,
  and it's pretty intense. It will build up your
  leg muscles like nothing else in the world
  (arms too), but be prepared for a serious
  investment of time and effort. Remember,
  this is an Olympic sport. I have friends that
  work the Renaissance Faire circuits (and
  choreograph Shakespeare and an occasional
  historical movie) and some that do actual
  swordfighting, and that's even more intense. There's quite a few groups out there
  that use naked steel without the tips, and
  weapons from rapiers to broadswords and
  full armor. You can usually find them in
  city parks or an offshoot of a fencing class.
  If you're an adventuresome sort, go for it.
  You'll meet interesting people and have a
  lot of fun. Make sure your medical insurance is paid up.

- Rock Climbing, and the Rock Gym. If you're
  not afraid of heights, this is good exercise
  (especially the arms and shoulders), but

this isn't for everyone, and you should be fairly fit before you start it. The rock-climbing walls are good practice, but if you're serious about this, you have to go to the rock itself – outside and with the accoutrements – ropes, pitons, boots, etc. Watch out for snakes and check your insurance again.

• Pilates – this is the grandmother of all floor exercise systems, focusing on the "core", your stomach and back muscles. If you want a flat stomach, this will do it, no question. Pilates "Reformer" classes are wonderful, if you have the dedication and the money. If you want to do it at home, buy a DVD and start in. You'll need a mat at the least, and lots of determination, but it's worth it. Pilates works like nothing else. Combine it with anything that gets you moving and on your feet as cardiovascular exercise and you've got a complete winner.

• Boxing. You have to be serious about getting in shape, and ready for some bruises, but maybe this appeals to you. Watch "Million Dollar Baby" before you start. Lots of women are doing this and loving it. The previous cautions are here, especially the insurance part. Also, be prepared for bruises and black eyes. Makeup will help with this. The speed bag is a bitch, trust me.

- Kickboxing. See above. I have a friend who is really into this, a 50-year-old who's amazing, in the best shape of anyone I've ever known. She got bored with karate after she got a black belt (see above, sigh). She really just liked the kicking and punching parts the best anyway, so she likes this a lot. Same cautions as last three above apply. Note: This is great for working out your aggressions and stress. Don't take it on the road, unless in extreme circumstances. If you get good at this, give some thought to anger management therapy if you want to enter dark alleys a lot for practice. Of course, I'm all about lowering the crime rate, so I'm a little ambivalent here.....exercise <u>and</u> social justice, hmmm.

- NIA – Neuromuscular integrative action. To me, this seems like a combination of dance, tai chi, yoga and martial arts, and what could be better than that? Fluid movements, good music, choreography, it provides both aerobic and strength movements for an overall great workout. NIA studios are opening everywhere, but you may have to search a bit. There's a website, www.nia-nia.com, which lists teachers and some basic history of the practice. It was designed by former aerobics instructors who were looking for a little more, well… fun, fluidity and music that didn't come from Three Dog Night or Richard Simmons. I haven't personally tried this, but friends that have swear by it. Don't be put off by the NIA people's somewhat airy-fairy attitude toward changing your life forever and just give it a try. Anyone can do this, you don't have to be in shape to start.

• Gyrokinesis and Gyrotonics – based on a combination of dance, yoga, tai-chi and Pilates moves, the gyro exercise systems are unique and different. They were developed by Juliu Horvath, a former ballet dancer who had an injury, and through physical therapy and learning a lot about different types of body movement therapies, including Feldenkrais, came up with these. Gyrokinesis is the baby of the two – the class usually starts on a stool, doing fluidic movements similar to yoga, and moves on to a mat, with more yoga-like exercises, but none are held for long. Gyrokinesis is easy to start, and is about movement – emphasizing circles, not lines, and fluidity. The gyrokinesis system is easy to start, and as you go, you'll develop the ability to do the exercises to the fullest if you stick with it. Gyrotonics is the fulfillment of this exercise system, utilizing weight machines that look a bit like medieval torture devices, but are uniquely designed. A lot of dancers and actors are doing this, and there's little doubt about its effectiveness for developing a long, lean, streamlined body. Gyrokinesis is pretty affordable, about $15-20 a class, but gyrotonics is a little pricier, sometimes $50 or more per class, and the equipment is quite expensive. Unless you've got a very large house, there's nowhere to put the con-traptions that's unobtrusive, (and I'm not sure you'd want to), going to the studio is the only option and it's a costly one over time. They also have DVDs, for the gyro-kinesis system, but once again, combine it with an aerobic activity. Go on line to look for studios near you, they are proliferating at a rapid rate, too.

You have options, never think you don't. I know there's lots of things I haven't included, but then I'm not into Nascar or wrestling either. There's some lines to be drawn in the interests of taste and common sense, I daresay. I didn't include swimming, because after all, this is common sense, and if you have a pool, you should have enough sense to be using it. Or a lake, the ocean, a pond, a river, if you live on or near one, get out there and get wet. If this has not occurred to you before, once again, get off the couch and into the water. These resources shouldn't be for landscaping purpos-es, or providing income for pool service people, they're meant to be used. Any movement you do is magnified ten times by the weight of the water itself so this is not only good sense, it's ten times good sense.

What did I say at the beginning of this chapter? Do something for a minimum of 30 minutes (an hour is better) at least five days out of seven that gets your heart rate up, your blood pumping and makes you feel alive. The truth is, once you give any exercise three days or more, it becomes a habit you won't want to give up, because you're already going to feel better, physically and mentally, practically instantly. Within two weeks you're going to see a difference, and within two months, that difference will be very pronounced.

Mix and match – tango one day a week, do yoga for two, aerobics for one, lift weights for one, Pilates for another. Variety, that's the real secret. Getting active is very addictive. You'll find out something very interesting happens once you start exercising at any of these things – one thing leads to another. It's amazing, and true.

I said it twice. Not saying it again. I've given you options plus. One or more of them is going to work for you, unless you're comatose, and I don't think that's true, if you read this far. Off your ass and onto your feet, darlings.

Chapter Seven
Great Good Food:
The Best, the Worst and Why

This has been hard, hasn't it? I'm sort of a bitch about things, telling you what to do, how to do it, and why you should. Why should you listen to me, anyway? I'm not perfect, any more than you are. I've made lots of mistakes, wasted time, and done a lot of stupid things in my quest for just plain looking good. But I've learned from those mistakes, the hard way, and then moved on to learn about nutrition, food and what the human body needs.

I discovered real food and the difference it makes, which is all the difference in the world. If there is a magic bullet for health, good food is that, combined with exercise.

I love feeling good, and it takes exercise in some form to make you feel really good physically. Once you start exercising regularly, you will be amazed at how good you feel, and you won't want to give it up because of the difference it makes in not only how you look, but how you feel – emotionally and mentally. I'll always remember a good friend, who told me at one point in my life when I was going through a bad time: "exercise every day and make yourself sweat, go outside and breathe fresh air, and love yourself" – the best advice I've ever received.

I am also very fond of looking good, and I do. But – if I don't eat right and exercise, I'll start looking and feeling like a glob of something Tyler Durden digs out of dumpsters. Also, buying clothes is a lot of fun when you look good wearing them, and when you're looking good, damn near anything looks good on you.

I am enormously disgusted with greedy people, whether they're the ones behind glossily packaged processed food, the many diet plans and programs that promise you'll look like a half-starved has-been actress if you pay them and follow their advice, so-called diet doctors and their know-it-all bestsellers, some cable TV exercise guru, Internet diet sites, the latest chi-chi exercise studio in town with some new and assuredly hip idea of what it takes to be slim and wonderful – all of whom profess to be "experts" in one field or another, but all of whom are really just trying to make a buck from other people's misery and desire to make their lives and their bodies better, selling bad advice and worse nutrition. With the huge amount of products and people pushing them in this world, I've learned to separate truth from fiction, and quality from what's being huckstered.

We all want the same thing – to be in the best shape we can, and it's not really just about how we look, but how we feel, how we live our lives every day and what makes us happy – and what makes us happy is all those things, and knowing that we're doing the best we can, by being informed and knowledgeable. Looking into the mirror and liking what you see is a great feeling and very achievable.

You've read this far, and now you know: it doesn't require trips to GNC, or Hi-Health and taking some weird protein powder, the latest tropical berry discovery, combining food groups and eating lots of alfalfa sprouts and dry chicken, running four miles in the rain, going to the latest Hollywood-style weight loss emporium, or the latest chic studio.

This isn't an instant weight loss program, although for some of you, it might be quicker than others. You're going to lose weight, and get healthier and fit, no question. How long it takes is variable. Be assured of this:

If you eat good food, eat less of it, and exercise, you will lose weight and get toned and fit. You are in control. Your mind and your body will be in tune, and this is something you will do for the rest of your life, because you'll love it and love what it's doing for you. You will find that it's automatic, that you KNOW, and you will want to live like this forever, and pass it on to those you care about. It's addictive, once you begin, and with this, that's a good thing.

I am deliberately not going to write Day One, Day Two meals and food lists, because I think you're smarter than that, and frankly it's boring and confining. You want to eat fresh food, cook it right, and think, in every social situation you are in, from expensive restaurants to family barbecues to pizza with the baseball team, about what's good for you. Remember everything you've read here and act accordingly.

At first, it may be helpful for you to make lists of what you are eating. Don't leave out anything, from that doughnut at 7 AM in the meeting, to the leftover pizza that was just sitting there in the refrigerator to the crab puffs you couldn't resist at the Chinese place. This way, you'll know where you need to get tough with yourself. Pretty soon, it'll be obvious that you have a problem passing a tray of high carb dumplings or the chocolate candy bowl, and you'll adjust your habits.

To help you along, here's lists of the food you want to start eating. I advise you to check your pantry and refrigerator and throw out (seriously) anything you might have on hand that doesn't fit into the following lists, and for god's sake don't buy any more crap, i.e., processed food, box dinners, frozen breakfast pastries, or succumb to fast foods, restaurants or social pressure at dinner parties where hostesses serve food you know you don't want to eat. Picky is good.

The lists below are more or less in order of impor-tance, with comments (of course, who are you dealing with here?) I may have overlooked a few things here and there, but in general, this will get you on the right track.

Buy food as close to the source as you can. Buy your food in the more natural food markets if you have them close by, i.e., Whole Foods, Sprouts, Wegman's, Trader Joe's, Fresh & Easy and others. If not, regular supermarkets have good food, too, just be careful and read the labels, and wash all produce well. (Don't be afraid of dirt – your food is grown in it, and it's the chemical pesticides you can't see that are dangerous.)

If I were to tell you the most perfect way to eat, I would have to tell you simply this: vegetables, and lots of them, fruit, ditto, and whole grains. Little meat, less dairy, watch the sugar and fats and a little olive oil to cook with. But, there's so much out there in food wonderland USA that we aren't going to ignore or give up, that we must be realistic, pragmatic and still make smart choices whenever we can.

Food isn't just fuel – it's memories, tradition, romance and tragedy, holidays, love, family and adventure. Come on, the only way you're going to think quinoa and fava beans every night are adventurous is if you've been in the Peace Corps way too long.

Even so, begin making the foundation of your food intake vegetables, fruit and whole grains. I'm going to start this list with the foods you should be eating the most of:

Vegetables

Tomatoes – I know, it's technically a fruit, but nobody really thinks of it that way. High in lycopene, which is super good for you, delicious in any form, fresh, pureed, made into marinara. EuroFresh, Campari and other brands sells smaller ones that you can get in most supermarkets that almost taste homegrown. Forget the pale tasteless big ones. Tomatoes are first on the list because they're something you should eat a lot of, and start our list with color. Good rule of thumb is the brighter and more colorful the vegetable, the better it is for you.

Red, yellow, orange bell peppers (green, too, but the others are tastier)

Onions– green, yellow, red

Leeks

Fresh garlic

Broccoli – great anti-oxidant, learn to love it

Spinach – full of iron

Eggplant

Beets

Peas – green, snap, sugar, sweet

Green beans – and yellow ones

Alfalfa sprouts

Artichokes

Asparagus

Carrots

Cucumbers

Brussels sprouts – sort of bitter, but try it with cheese sauce

Mushrooms – all of them

Lettuce – romaine, butter, leaf, red, anything but iceberg, which has zero nutritional value, avoid it completely

Squash – acorn, spaghetti, zucchini, banana, all

Yams and sweet potatoes (they are different)

Radishes

Bok Choy – and check Asian markets, they have lots of wonderful veggies you aren't familiar with, but are excellent, and really tasty

Cauliflower

Radishes

Cabbage

Potatoes – go with red, they're best for you, and leave the skins on.

Celery

Chiles

Corn – remember it's starchy and somewhat hard to digest

There's others, lots of new field greens and lettuces, and roots, like turnips and rutabagas, which are all right but starchy. I always like to try vegetables I'm not familiar with, you never know. With cooked vegetables, think about lemon juice, and a little garlic for flavoring, instead of butter.

Fruits

Apples

Bananas (lots of potassium)

Blueberries – the best anti-oxidant

Blackberries – great anti-oxidant

Pomegranates – the same

Strawberries

Raspberries

Peaches

Nectarines

Pears

Avocados – fatty, but monosaturated fatty, and full of omega-3 acids, very good

Grapes

Apricots

Figs

Dates

Cranberries

Grapefruit

Oranges, Tangerines, Tangelos

Melons – watermelon, cantaloupe, honeydew and more

Kiwi

Lemons

Limes

Papayas

Plums

Grains, Pasta, Beans, Rice, Nuts

Rice

Brown is best. It takes longer to cook, and takes some getting used to, if all you've eaten is plain white rice, but it's very good for you, has lots more nutrients and less calories. Once you get used to real rice, you won't care for the white pap anymore, really. Wild rice is great as well, same thing. If you must have white rice, go with jasmine or basmati. They both have good texture, fragrance and taste and they only take 15 minutes to cook. Rice that takes a minute to cook, or has a bunch of chemicals and flavorings are not your friends, if you value your waistline and your taste buds.

Flour

Unbleached white flour. Never eat regular white flour again, for lots of reasons: all the nutrients are gone, and it's bleached out with chlorine and chemicals, yuck. You can use unbleached flour in any recipe that calls for white flour, including cakes, and it works just fine, I don't care what the recipes say. I don't know why they sell this stuff – it must be a hangover from people reading "Heidi" and wanting white rolls like the "rich people" have. The peasants had it right all the time. (Just to let you know how pervasive this sort of thing is, I did see an article in the weekend magazine of the Sunday paper not long ago that extolled the virtues of bleached flour when making pancakes. The cook/writer who wrote this obviously needs psychotherapy, and I wouldn't want to have breakfast at his house. He's probably serving ground puppy sausage too, because it's tender.)

Then, branch out, go with Red Mill, they make excellent flours – oat, whole wheat, buckwheat, ground flaxseed, etc. Tip: keep flour in your freezer and you'll never get weevils or bugs in it.

Take a walk on the wild side, get adventurous and go with falafel, quinoa, millet, couscous, buckwheat, tabbouleh. Buckwheat pancakes are the best thing ever, my grandfather used to make them when I was little, and they were fabulous.

This gets us into bread, that staple of life in America. I love bread, it's the best ever. But here's the thing: if you're going to buy bread for sandwiches, spend the money and get the good stuff. If you see rainbows or colored dots, move on. Cutting up artisan bread every morning is a pain, but tasty and you have to buy it fresh every day – so for some modicum of convenience, go with a good, tasty grain bread. Try them out, see what you like and stick with it. For sandwiches, Oroweat's Oatnut is great, as is Women's Bread, a little harder to find, and very expensive. But then, you don't want to eat a lot of it anyway, do you?

For anything else, artisan-type whole loaf breads baked fresh are the best, whether it's peasant-style white, sourdough, olive, garlic/rosemary, asiago cheese, a hundred other variations – crusty on the outside and soft inside. Steer clear of those "fresh out of the oven French bread" things in supermarkets, they're just unsliced warm Rainbo bread. Supermarkets are getting smarter about bread and you can find some pretty good artisan bread in supermarket bakeries lately.

Cereal

Most of the big commercial cereal makers start with ingredients that have had all the nutrient value sucked out of them and then they add back in all sorts of "vitamins and minerals", along with lots of things I can't pronounce. Lucky Charms and that creepy leprechaun is a big no, but you weren't expecting me to say yes on that one, were you? Sorry, so is just about every other heavily advertised cereal on the planet. If it has coupons in the Sunday paper, you can figure it's not for you. Tony the Tiger, Captain Crunch and their friends are not your friends, like lots of others you'd least expect, for instance the good old Quaker oatman – that hat he wears makes you think he's holy and wholesome but this guy's gone to the dark side (read Madison Avenue) except for his plain old rolled oats. If you check the caloric intake on the label of Quaker granola, your eyes will spin. Oatmeal is great – and yes, steel cut Irish oats are awesome, if you have the time to make them in the morning. If not, try old fashioned oatmeal, because you can microwave a small portion very quickly, (as fast as the instant stuff) and add in some brown sugar or honey and milk, and it's pretty darn good, and good for you. Or, try making your own granola, it's not hard and it's pretty tasty, too. (I've got a recipe later).

Pasta

Who doesn't love pasta? But sparingly, unless you want to look like Tony Soprano. He didn't get that gut from the marinara sauce. Steer clear of plain old white flour pasta, and that usually means the trusty old American brands. Whole wheat pasta comes in a lot of varieties, but my favorite is multi-grain. This combines best taste and healthy all in one, it's great. The other secret is angel hair pasta. You can use this in any recipe that calls for spaghetti or linguine, and it folds oh so nicely around a fork, instead of that big fat noodle or hefty flat one. If you've got the time and the equipment, try making your own. The difference is remarkable, and it's a lot of fun.

Beans

Learn to love beans. They are chock-full of protein and no fat. People are afraid to eat beans because they're afraid they'll fart, and yes, that's a side effect to some degree. However, it's not that bad, especially if you soak them and put a little baking soda in while that's happening. You can use them in salads, main dishes and soups and they're wonderful.

Lentils

Chickpeas (garbanzo)

Great Northern beans (the big white ones)

Navy beans (somewhat smaller)

White beans (smallest)

Cannelli beans

Black beans

Lima beans

Pinto beans

Refried beans, especially the vegetarian ones, because they're made without lard

Split peas

Kidney beans

Soybeans (Edamame, Chinese restaurants first discovered steaming these and selling them as a side dish and they're gotten very popular)

Tofu

Made from soybeans, I find cooking tofu works best "extra firm". This is practically a whole 'nother category, when you get to Thai and Chinese food especially. You can substitute tofu for meat in any recipe. My favorite Chinese restaurant does tofu cut into triangles, about 1/4 " thick, stir-fried with fresh veggies and different sauces, and people order this six times more than any meat, it's so crispy and good. (Check the recipe section for the secrets.) Andrew Weil, MD, has extolled its virtues (anti-cancer, anti-aging, etc.) much better than I can, check out his many books, he's the best.

I have a friend who makes smoothies with silken tofu, and these are really good. Blenders are wonderful things. Invest in a good one, you'll be glad you did.

However, I have a caveat on soy: it's being marketed by the food industry as the best thing for you since sliced bread (and we all know how that one went.) I suspect there's an agricultural surplus here. Eating too much soy for some people can cause digestive problems, so be aware of that. Once again, I have to go with my grandfather: moderation in all things.

Nuts

Almonds (super anti-oxidant)

Cashews

Walnuts

Peanuts

Coconut

Flaxseed (super anti-oxidant)

Macadamia nuts

Pine nuts

Pumpkin seeds

Sunflower seeds

Soy nuts

Pecans

Nut butters: if you grew up on peanut butter, (and who didn't, I still love a P&J sandwich, except in brown bag lunches, where something weird happens to it after four hours), you're thinking just peanut butter, most likely Jif or Peter Pan. However, these peanut butters are filled with things not so good for you, first off, high fructose corn syrup. Move on. Try almond or cashew butter, super good for you, high in anti-oxidants, and tastes fabulous, especially on toast. Trust me on this, it's yummy. Or try natural peanut butter, without the corn syrup and chemicals.

Dairy

Now, this is tricky. We've all grown up with and been conditioned to think that milk, butter, cheese, eggs and anything made from these things is good for you, and coming from the right source, they are. Thank the American Dairy Council, they've got a very big advertising budget. Remember those cheesy ads with famous celebrities displaying their milk moustaches? Oh please, those botoxed lips probably haven't really touched milk in many a moon. It's amazing how money can distort people's sense of reality. However, ask any vascular surgeon or nutritionist and you're going to hear the truth. Cheese babies are fatso babies and heavy cheese-consuming adults are going to be surgery candidates sooner or later. A vascular surgeon I know always passed on the free pizza brought in by the big drug company lunches and called those who did indulge "my next patients waiting to happen".

As for good old milk, it's been processed half to death. Once again, the food industry and the government, always looking out for us, have sold us quite a bill of goods when it comes to pasteurization and homogenization. You won't die or get a disease from drinking whole milk that's organic, unpasteurized, or raw. For further information on this, please read Nina Planck's <u>Real Food</u>, and google the Weston Price website.

At the very least, do buy organic dairy products. They don't have the hormones and other nasty things that are in corporate produced dairy. Trader Joe's again is good, as well as other organic markets, and even the usual ones, if you read the labels.

Yogurt

Great, try for organic, but read the labels, and even better, make your own. This was fashionable back in the 70s, and it's making a comeback.

Cheese

We all love it, but in moderation. Most commercial cheese is not so good. Try feta, goat cheese, Stilton, gorgonzola, asiago, fontina, Jarlsberg. Cheese is a gift from cows and goats and we shouldn't ignore it. Cheese with real flavor allows you to use less of it. Branch out, there's a lot out there besides Kraft slices (plastic and horrible). Go to a good market and test out cheeses you never heard of, you're going to be surprised and delighted.

Every time I go to a Mexican restaurant and see somebody ordering cheese enchiladas I'm tempted to give them a vascular surgeon friend's card, or at least recommend a better place to eat. The yellow stuff they're slurping up is clogging their arteries as they swallow. Yikes. Needless to say, most Mexican eateries don't enjoy seeing me anymore, could be the look of horror on my face.

Eggs

Well, we covered this before. Since you know about eggs now, I don't have to say it again, do I?

Butter

OK, it's a fat. But, it's a lot better than margarine made out of who knows what, (NEVER eat that stuff) and sometimes you have to use it, because there's just nothing else that will do. Just use half of what you used to, and don't ever slather it on fresh cooked veggies, please.

Meat, Poultry, Fish

Especially in America, we've all been conditioned once again to think that a roast on the table, turf 'n surf for the ultimate date dinner, and a chicken in the pot means things are going very well indeed. You can afford meat every night, your date's not a cheapskate, and times are good. It's comforting, and it's traditional. Hmm. Not so much.

Not eating some kind of meat every day is a difficult concept to wrap your mind around, even when you consciously know differently, because conditioning is one tough cookie. You know it's really not good for you, it's fat and calorie laden at its best, but somehow the "good life" is associated with having as much of it as you like, from prime rib to Sloppy Joes to But-terballs.

Remember when you toyed around with becoming a vegetarian in 9th grade and your mother freaked? "You'll get anemic, you won't grow, you'll die an early death" was mine's mantra and eventually I just gave in. I think mostly it was she didn't want to deal with my father's attitude or cooking anything radically different, because the neighbors would think we'd just turned Muslim or he wasn't doing so well career-wise.

Then there's supermarkets, advertising and restaurants. That huge section that usually runs across the whole back of the store is filled with meat. Every holiday means Easter ham, Thanksgiving turkey, Christmas prime rib, 4th of July fried chicken.

Nobody thinks Labor Day shrimp or Halloween falafel, or birthday halibut. When's the last time you saw an ad for a restaurant that talked about its salads (unless McDonald's was trying to make you think it was a health food place?) Or, a restaurant that was famous for its broccoli? Not likely.

Sensible eating means you use moderation in all things, especially meat. You aren't going to get anemic, have no energy, need B-12 shots or any other silly thing. You are going to lose weight and be healthier.

Red meat

Beef, pork, lamb, veal. Try to buy this as "hormone-free", or organic, and as lean as you can. I highly recommend finding a local rancher and getting a quarter, half or a "box" of natural grass-fed beef. You can buy your other meats this way as well. Eat this no more than once a week, or on special occasions. (The filet mignon date night, or beef taco fiesta night, you get the drift.) I personally rarely eat beef and when I do, it's local grass-fed Angus. The USDA does NOT test for Ecoli in commercial beef, unless you count one cow out of a million, which aren't good odds to me. As we discussed earlier, government agencies are not your friends and they aren't looking out for your best interests, but those of the meat industry.

Chicken, turkey

Again, go for "free range, organic" if you can. Try substituting ground turkey breast for beef in meat loaf, lasagna, tacos, and other things and you'll find it's really good. It's leaner and much better for you.

Fish and Shellfish

Don't give me that old "I hate fish" or "I'm allergic" routine. Lots of us started that one back in the day when our fathers caught anything that was dumb enough to hit their lines. Dinner that night was usually fried something from the water that had enough bones in it to make a miniature T Rex. Arghh. (Mom was on hand with French bread, saying things like "It'll wash down the bones so they don't get caught in your throat." Double arrgh compounded with fear, always a good dietary suggestion.) I have to admit it was local, and organic, though.

Then you discovered lobster and shrimp and knew all fish wasn't boney and fried and you rejoiced, didn't you? Moving on from there, to the wondrous taste of halibut, monkfish, ahi tuna and salmon, to say nothing of abalone, scallops and clams – well, the seaworld's your oyster – pun intended. I caution you about a few things:

- canned tuna. We've all been trained to think white tuna is the greatest, but it's also highest in mercury and contaminates. Instead, go with light tuna. It's got a better flavor anyway, but it's harder to find in real chunk form lately. Look for tuna fillet, or "gourmet" chunk light tuna packed in olive oil – don't buy the watery junk they're selling as "light chunk tuna". The packing of tuna has changed – there must be a cost-cutting measure in effect at Starkist and Chicken of the Sea, or they're trying to train us now to go with the foil packets. Sigh – once again, marketing and profit takes a front seat to taste.

- Go with wild salmon, not farm-raised. It's harder to find, but try Trader Joe's frozen, depends on the time of year. At the market, ask the fish guy/butcher if the salmon is wild. They may not know why it's better, but they'll know which kind they've got.

- Always smell fresh fish. It shouldn't be rankly fishy-smelling or slimy to the touch. Supermarkets especially tend to sell older fish. Go to a fish market if you have one nearby.

- In restaurants, the "catch of the day" is wildly variant. A top-notch restaurant with a chef who is really savvy buys "first catch", where the fishermen come back early in the morning to ship their first catch, FedExed out to restaurants that insist upon it, but the usual standard is the fish that comes back at the end of the day, also shipped out daily, but it's been sitting in the hold all day, and the restaurant doesn't get it until the next morning, really. Major difference.

Sweeteners

Sugar:

Buy cane sugar, not beet, it's just better-tasting. A few cents more, but once again, you get what you pay for. Brown sugar is better, but any sugar at all is going to cost you, so be careful.

Honey:

Lots of different sources are what give each type of honey its unique and wonderful taste. There's orange blossom, clover, all sorts of other flowers and plants. Pick one that you like best. Yum.

Syrups:

Pure maple syrup is the only one I recommend. All the other pancake syrups, even those old favorite brands and cute bottles, are mostly high fructose corn syrup with flavorings.

Anything else is pretty much some manufactured sort of thing. I advocate staying as far away from these as you can, and the list includes aspartame, sucralose (marketed as Splenda), and saccharine. There's a lot of testing that's been done, and the government declares that all of them are safe, but you take your chances on this, I think. Aspartame in particular bothers me a lot, since it's a byproduct that was discovered to be sweet by accident, and the jury's still out on exactly what it does inside the human body. Sucralose is another one – it's really a chlorocarbon, manufactured because of you and the trillions of dollars the diet and food industry make from selling it. Some things take many years to show up in the "not good for you" side of things, so I figure better safe than sorry. I'm still waiting for the headlines one morning, "Aspartame causes brain damage" or "sucralose causes liver calcification". Might never happen, but just in case, I'm not eating anything that has it.

Fats and Oils

There's really only one oil you should be using:

Olive oil – extra virgin. It works for everything, from making salad dressing to cooking. OK, it's a little more expensive than all the others, but it's worth it.

If you're having a fondue party, invest in peanut oil, it works better for long term heating.

For damn near anything else, it's olive oil, no question. There's other oils, like walnut, sesame, macadamia, flaxseed (fabulously good for you), oils that have many uses, and by all means, use them. But for everyday use, it's olive oil. The only exception I make to this is if you're doing fondue. Peanut oil works better, it's just that simple.

If you have vegetable, canola or corn oil, etc., use it up or throw it out. Canola oil is a weird one. It's touted as the oil of choice, but its history is damning. It's really rapeseed oil, but the media figured who would buy anything with "rape" in its name, and they were right. It used to be used for industrial purposes, and wasn't refined for human consumption. It still can't be used in infant formula, so think about that. It's a profiteer's and marketer's dream, and that always makes me shy away. If it's that good, how come it has to be concealed behind another name and lots of advertising? Check it out on www.wikipedia.com and come to your own conclusions. I don't think you'll be eating anything cooked it in real soon.

I realize I've sort of bypassed the vegetable short-ening thing. For making pie crusts, cookies, and pretty much baking all those yummy all-American desserts we grew up on, you have to make some hard choices. Most of these recipes let you use butter, so try that. It tends to bake faster, so keep that in mind or you might have some black bottom chocolate chip cookies. For pie crust, this is difficult. Make an exception here. Or, just don't eat these things anymore, but as always, this is your choice. NEVER eat store-bought processed bak-ery goods, they're loaded with more preservatives and compounds than a high school chemistry class. Then there's lard. It's animal fat. Just the word "lard" sort of says it all, doesn't it? However, properly rendered, I understand it's not as terrible for you as it sounds. Makes great piecrust and tortillas, too.

Beverages, Drinks

Water, water water.

If you have good tap water, you are blessed. Many places in America don't, and that's a sad but true fact. In the city I live in, the tap water tastes of chlorine and mold and other things that remind me of "Day of the Living Dead". (Just for kicks, one morning I used the pool chlorine tester on my tap water, and the tap water was higher in chlorine than the pool I'd just put chlorine in. Pretty scary.) Even the coffee tastes horrible made with it.

So, you have choices: a good filtration system hooked up in-house, one of those on your kitchen faucet things, a Brita filter pitcher, or bottled water, an industry that I wish I'd bought stock in, because it's going crazy. (It's also making one hell of an environmental cleanup mess. So buy the big ones. I've taken to washing and refilling some of my water bottles from the Brita pitcher, so I feel a little better, and I recycle.) However, keep in mind that bottled water comes in many guises:

- The supermarket house brand, or some other semi-local supplier. Sometimes this isn't bad, but remember that it's most likely just filtered tap water.

- The mountain spring water kinds, like Arrowhead, and lots of other local imitators, who like to make you think it's from snowmelt at the head of some pristine mountain river (and those are where in America these days?) Maybe so, but think about it.

- Evian, Perrier, Fiji, Pellegrino, Voss, any others that cost a lot. These are great tasting waters, no doubt about it, and I tend to trust most of their claims and bottling. But you're going to pay for it. Besides, I keep wondering how the Fiji Islands have an endless supply of artesian water or when those European glaciers are going to melt. Call me skeptical.

I've listed these in order of cost, from low to high. If you can afford it, go with the last one. If not, taste and decide. Personally, I use Brita filtered water for everything I cook, from coffee to rice, and drink Fiji because I like its taste and it's convenient to carry around. I know, you're thinking, water's water, is she nuts? Try it, and decide for yourself.

Sodas, Frozen Drink Mixes, Fruit and Vegetable Juices

Soda is junk in any form – regular or diet. Almost all the big soda manufacturers use high fructose corn syrup for sweeteners, not sugar in all the regular sodas they make. This stuff isn't good for you, on any level – nutritionally, economically, (or socially, but that's another book….) Then, if you go for diet, trying to feel good about yourself, think again: it's mostly aspartame, or sucralose and we've already talked about that stuff. There's also a nasty aftertaste. Hansen's is better, and other "natural" soda manufacturers that still use sugar – if you're close to the Mexican border, you can actually find bottled sodas that have sugar, instead of high fructose corn syrup. Still, it's a lot of extra calories that you don't need just for sake of hydrating. Stick to water or teas instead.

Watch out for supermarket label drinks like "raspberry-peach flavored sparkling water" which has artificial flavors and sweeteners like aspartame, and watch the bottled "teas" because these can be filled with weird ingredients.

Drink mixes, especially the dry ones, have so many nasty things, and usually aspartame as a sweetener, that I can't recommend any of them. Anything with "country" in the label is usually really awful-tasting and should be avoided like the plague.

Frozen juices are almost always made with high fructose corn syrup, even Minute Maid, which I always trusted as a kid. How disappointing and disillusioning that was. Check the labels.

Fruit and vegetable bottled juices: Most of this is made from "concentrate" and lots of other things. Check the labels once again, sigh. The brands you have always trusted are sometimes full of junk. Go for the ones that say "organic" or natural fruit and vegetable juices. There are some out there, but you have to read the labels. Don't freak out because it says "sugar". Sugar is natural, and how much you drink of it is your choice. At least it's organic, real, and not giving you some disease that shows up in 20 years. I still like V-8. Tip: when you have a cold, go for tomato juice, not just orange juice. When you have muscle aches, especially knees, try pineapple juice, it's made from a bromeliad, which cuts inflammation.

Alcohol

Wine: So far, it looks as though it's true: having one or two glasses of wine a day is good for you. Absolutely. Good wine is a gift from the gods. They've discovered that white's almost as good as red, by the way, just doesn't have reservato. Grapes are wonderful things.

Get wine that you like, experiment, and develop a palate. It's not as mysterious as wine aficionados make it sound. You'll be surprised at how soon you'll be able to discern good from not so good, and it goes on from there. Remember that price does make a difference, but there's bargains to be had. Stay away from boxes (we used to call it "teacher wine", sorry, my old colleagues, or the large size bottles), and make the acquaintance of the people at a good wine store, their advice is usually invaluable – but don't be intimidated if there's a snotty wine store clerk, the only reason he knows anything is because he probably steals five bottles a week and will be fired by the owner soon.

Once you know, you can shop the supermarket, they always have sales on good wine. Another caveat here: organic wine is on the rise, because it doesn't have added sulfites. Sulfites are used as a preservative and lots of people get headaches, stuffy noses, and other side effects from them. Organic wine doesn't use them, or pesticides on their grapes. If you have any of the aforementioned problems, try organic wine.

Liquor: Well, not so sure it's good for you, any of it. But – keep in mind that a mint julep is said to cure anything viral, (not to mention the old Indian remedy of lemon, whiskey and sugar – drink enough of it and you'll feel better or at least not remember why you were sick in the first place.) And then there's martinis, cosmopolitans and margueritas,which certainly have their place. Think of it this way: you know what you can handle, and you know it certainly has caloric value, as well as a sneaky way of putting on weight that's hard to lose, especially around the middle.

That's it. I'm sure I've missed a few of your favorites, or you have questions I didn't answer. But, read again before you email me. You have to think for yourself a bit on this one. If you've been paying attention, you know what you should be eating and drinking by now, so don't ask me stuff like "If I use cool whip, does that matter?" or "can I use scalloped potatoes in the box when I'm in a hurry?" Come on.

Remember, I'm not telling you to change everything you hold dear. I respect tradition as much as you, maybe more. My mom's cherry pie will forever hold a special place in my heart, and I know how to make it, and enjoy it. That's not the point of all this. Knowing is the point. I also know even if my mom used vegetable shortening, she sure as hell didn't use sucralose ("even good for baking!")

Chapter Eight
Creativity Really Is
The Spice of Life:
A Few Fabulous Recipes,
Cookbooks and Roadmaps
to Get You Started

I'm not taking you through days of breakfast, lunch and dinner, because I think that by now, you've figured this out for yourself. <u>Make it a rule to only eat exactly what you want</u> – not something that looks iffy just because somebody brings it in to work, or serves it at a dinner or buffet, or because you're hungry and it'll do until something better comes along. Don't make a big deal out of it, but start being picky. Once you get used to eating fresh, quality food, you'll find you have no trouble tactfully declining anything that isn't.

Also, food suggestions in diet books annoy me, because I don't really want to have egg whites and wheat toast for breakfast, or a can of drained tuna dumped on a cracker for lunch, and a dry chicken breast with steamed broccoli for dinner. The "recipes" section in most diet books usually involve bulgar wheat or some incredibly nasty-tasting recipe for lima beans, and always involve lemons and garlic on everything instead of a great-tasting sauce or dressing. I'm sure if lemons and garlic could talk and carry knives, they'd be organizing a revolution. They deserve better.

What follows are some recipes that I've created or stumbled onto through the years – that provide maximum taste and flavor with maximum pretty darn good nutrition and less fat. Remember these are suggestions, not diet recipes. You're not going to lose ten pounds in a week on these recipes, (you will do so eventually) but you will like them and hopefully incorporate them into your life, because they taste good, and they're good for you. If you like them, fine. If you don't, use your own, or start reading some cookbooks to find some you do.

Remember: eat good food that you like, and if it's not as low in calories as it could be, eat less of it. Enjoy food, don't ever eat tasteless pap just because it's supposed to be "good for you" or low in calories.

Just so we're very very clear on this, you're never going to lose ten pounds in a week on any diet or recipes, because even if you starve yourself and just drink chicken broth or water for seven days, any weight you lose you're going to put right back on. Anyone who tells you differently needs to seek out a good psychotherapist, or come over to my house so I can kick their ass. However, once you start eating real food, cooked well, and less of it, you will lose weight. That's the plain truth.

So, let's get started. I'm putting these in a sort of order of the day, but these are suggestions, not the holy grail. You have a life, and impromptu invitations and indulgences are the glue that holds life together.

Breakfast

This meal is often ignored, and shouldn't be. It tends to run the gamut from eggs/bacon/potatoes to half a grapefruit and dry toast to just coffee. I've heard the old "if I eat breakfast, I'm starving by 11" excuse, but once your body gets used to good food early in the day, you'll find you eat less at lunch and have more energy.

I've mentioned oatmeal, especially steel-cut oats, before, or one egg, one piece of toast and some fruit, or one of these options:

Bran Flaxseed Muffins

These are especially good for you, because flaxseed is sooo good for you. It's a super antioxidant, lowers bad cholesterol and is all around one of the best foods you can eat. These muffins are yummy, and if you store them in a container in the fridge, you'll have them all week.

1-1/2 cups unbleached white flour
3/4 cup Bob's Red Mill Flaxseed Meal
3/4 cup Bob's Red Mill Oat Bran flour
1 cup brown sugar
2 t. baking soda
1 t. baking powder
2 t. cinnamon
3 apples, medium sized, peeled and shredded (Granny Smith's are good)
3/4 cup milk
2 eggs
1 t. vanilla

You can add shredded carrots, raisins, currants as well. Just decrease the amount of apples accordingly.

Mix together first 7 ingredients, stir in apples, milk, eggs and vanilla. Mix together. It will be a bit lumpy, but that's OK. Fill muffin cups 3/4 full. This should make about a dozen. Use a good non-stick muffin pan, and I lightly grease it with olive oil. Bake at 350 degrees for about 18 minutes.

Thanks to Bob's Red Mill for the basics of this recipe.

Homemade Granola

This doesn't take long to make, tastes great and keeps well in an airtight container, too. As cereal it's fine, and even better mixed with yogurt, and fruit, and even makes a great snack.

There are lots of different choices you can make in the recipe:

Preheat oven to 275 degrees. Bake on middle rack (bottom one makes it too brown).

4 cups rolled oats (oldfashioned)

1 cup nuts: I like slivered almonds and cashews, mixed 1/2 and 1/2. (Experiment with others, too: macadamia, walnuts, sunflower seeds, etc.)

3/4 cup shredded coconut

1/2 cup dark brown sugar

1 t. cinnamon

1/4 cup wheat germ

1/4 olive oil

1/4 honey (you can try maple syrup instead if you like)

1 t. vanilla

1-1/2 cups dried cranberries, cherries or raisins. (Experiment here with other dried fruits if you like)

Mix together first six ingredients in large bowl. In a measuring cup, put oil, honey, vanilla. (You can heat this a little in the microwave to make it more liquid).

Stir together until well blended and spread in a large baking pan with sides.

Bake 35-45 minutes, depending on how brown you prefer, stirring and turning every 10 minutes or so. Remove from oven, stir in fruit and let cool. Store in airtight containers, up to 10 days, or freeze some, keeps for two months or so.

Note on granola: I've seen granola recipes that bake at 250 degrees, and for a longer time, say an hour and a half. Experiment if your oven is hot or it's getting too brown for your taste.

Vendetta Eggs

There was a movie a while back called "V for Vendetta" with Natalie Portman. It was interesting, but what I really remember about it was the breakfast that V served on our heroine's first day with him, so I tried it. It goes like this:

Take a slice of bread (I really like Oroweat's Oatnut for this). Cut a hole in the middle of it, about 2-1/2" in diameter. Butter both sides of the bread like you're making a grilled cheese sandwich. (Yeah, I know but olive oil just doesn't work for this.) Place in pan, turn on to medium high. When the butter melts on the bottom, crack one egg into the hole. Wait a bit, until it's browning, then flip over. Brown the other side. (You may have to experiment with this, depending on if you like your eggs easy, medium, or hard). Plate and enjoy. You can even eat this one on the run, if you cooked it medium or hard. Everybody I've ever made these for loves them.

Fruit Smoothies

Your options here are practically limitless with choices of fruit, yogurt, juices. These are absolutely yummy. I always put in a couple of tablespoons of flax-seed meal or wheat germ, too. Using fresh frozen fruit makes it really easy to keep stuff on hand. Here's my favorite:

1/2 banana
1/2 a small carton of vanilla yogurt
1/2 a small can of pineapple juice
Small handfuls of: strawberries, blueberries, sliced peaches, sliced mangoes
Put in blender and blend until liquefied. Wow.

Lunch and Dinner

Depending on your lifestyle, i.e., working or not, at home or not, children or not, lunch and dinner is all about what works for you. I'm a devotee of the family dinner, if you have one, not just for food, but for communication as well. People always used to eat their biggest meal of the day at lunch (and call it "dinner" if they lived on farms or ranches) because they were physically laboring. This isn't such a bad idea, even now, because we tend to be more sedentary in general, and still have less time to digest or work off a large meal if it's eaten in the evening. If you have children at home, though, this can be tricky, because they are always hungry, don't eat very well at lunch as a rule (take note and try some new lunchtime packing instead of that glop they serve at schools, good food isn't just for you, after all), and are conditioned to think "dinner" is the main meal of the day. So are you, but I did mention this was about changing your conditioned thinking, didn't I?

So, here's just a few recipes I've tried, modified and come to call my own from various sources and restaurants, as well as some I just made up over the years for food I love. Not all of them are particularly low-fat or low calorie, but they are all made with good ingredients, free from additives and not processed. These are not difficult, time-consuming, 50-ingredient, check-the-cookbook 20 times recipes, because I find that tedious and usually not worth the effort. They are, however, real crowd-pleasers, sometimes impressive, and most of all, yummy.

Appetizers

Bruschetta

Start with a good bread, fresh pane with a hard crust. Slice fairly thin, and brush with olive oil. Toast in oven, for five minutes, at 350 degrees. Remove from oven, spoon on a mixture of:

Finely chopped tomatoes
Minced garlic
Chopped fresh basil

Drizzle with a really good balsamic vinegar. You're done, enjoy.

There's a lot of variations possible here – mascarpone and sliced pears, salmon and capers, brie with sliced apples and drizzled honey – use your imagination. But this is the original. My only variation is roasted garlic, sliced, rather than minced. A restaurant I love serves this on a plank, and you can choose three or four different varieties. Add in a fruit plate, a good chardonnay, and you can call it dinner…..

Hummus

3 cups canned chickpeas, drained
2 t. salt
5 garlic cloves, minced
1/2 c tahini (sesame paste)
Juice of 3 lemons

Place all ingredients in Cuisinart with blade and process until fairly mashed. If it's too thick, add 3 T. water or more, to desired consistency. If you like it plain, fine. If not, you can add all sorts of seasonings and spices, use your imagination. Serve with pita bread or crackers.

Main Dishes

Raven's Marinara Sauce

This stuff is fabulous. You can use it for any pasta dish from fettuccine to lasagna, or pizza, or for just about anything else you can dream up. This makes enough for more than one meal, so I divvy it up and freeze it. If you're doing it, you might as well do it all at once, I think. Gives you options later. Yes, I do use canned crushed tomatoes. If you're really a purist, you can crush six pounds of fresh tomatoes by hand like they do in small hillside Italian villages. I have done it both ways, your choice as always.

8-10 cloves fresh garlic, minced
One onion, chopped
One pound sliced mushrooms
1/4 cup olive oil
One very large can crushed style tomatoes (Costco or Sam's Club has them), around 6 pounds.
Or, four big cans, (about 28 oz. each) crushed tomatoes
Chopped fresh basil
1/4 cup sugar (cuts the acidity of the tomatoes)
1/4 cup red wine (I like Merlot, but whatever you have about the house will work)
½ cup (or more if you like) grated Parmesan, asiago, reggiano or any hard Italian cheese

Sauté the garlic, onions, mushrooms in the olive oil. Add the tomatoes, basil, sugar and wine. Cook, stirring occasionally, for at least an hour or more, it lets the flavors blend. Towards the end blend in the cheese and let simmer.

Use immediately, or cool and refrigerate or freeze. Keeps for a few days in the refrigerator. You can add meatballs, Italian sausage or anything else you like – sometimes I add yellow or orange chopped bell peppers to the first part. You'll never buy spaghetti sauce in a jar again. (Sorry, Paul.) This is easy to make, cheaper, and oh so much better!

Turkey Meat Loaf

Yeah, OK, sue me. But, I was born in the Midwest, and this is a staple of life back there. I was embarrassed to admit to being a meat loaf fan before I worked this out. Serve it with a hunter mushroom sauce and garlic parmesan mashed red potatoes and it'll fly off the plates.

1 c. chopped onions
2 T. olive oil
1/3 c. chicken broth
2 T marinara sauce (or ketchup if you don't have any on hand)
2 T. Worcestershire sauce
Salt, pepper
2 lb. ground turkey breast
2 eggs
3/4 c. Italian bread crumbs

Sauté the onions in a little olive oil first, (sometimes I add some thin sliced mushrooms here, too). Add broth, sauces and stir. Take off heat and let cool for a minute or two.

Then, mix with the turkey, eggs and breadcrumbs, form a loaf and bake at 350 degrees for hour or so. To double this for a larger group, bake maybe 1/2 half an hour longer. I've found turkey takes a little longer to bake than ground beef, but it's worth it. If you like, you can top with ketchup and sprinkled brown sugar before you bake. This meat loaf has great flavor and is much better for you, to say nothing of better taste. Also makes great sandwiches.

Pan-sautéed Fish Filets

Start with fresh cod or halibut filets, about one inch think. Wash and pat dry. Heat 2 T olive oil in pan on medium-high heat, and sprinkle seasonings on the oil. Add fish, and add more seasoning to the top of the fish. Cook about 4-5 minutes on each side. Simple and great. You can use dill, oregano, lemon juice, garlic, pepper – get creative.

You can also use a mixture of balsamic vinegar and Dijon mustard, about 2T of each, mixed together. Heat the olive oil, add fish, and then put half the vinegar/mustard mix on top, and after turning, add the other half.

I also cook fresh scallops just this way, and sometimes serve them over a salad of fresh greens, with mandarin oranges, sliced water chestnuts and vinaigrette.

Thai Chicken (Swimming Rama)

This recipe is one I created after having this dish in a Seattle Thai restaurant. It's absolutely delicious. It looks complicated, but it's not, the hardest part is making the sauce, and that's not too daunting. I'm not giving quantities because you can make as much or little as you want, for one to many, with the chicken, spinach and rice. It comes in four parts:

Chicken breasts

Baby spinach leaves

Jasmine rice

Peanut sauce

Sauté chicken breasts in olive oil, with a little garlic, kosher salt and pepper until lightly browned. Remove from heat and slice into strips for manageability.

Peanut sauce recipe:

2 t olive oil

1/2 c minced onion, and 2 cloves minced garlic

1/2 c peanut butter, creamy or chunky

3 T brown sugar

1/2 t cayenne pepper (or more if you want it really hot)

1 t paprika

1 c coconut milk (look for in Asian food section)

1 t cornstarch, mixed into 1 T water

1 t lime juice

Sauté the onions and garlic in oil, reduce heat to medium. Add the peanut butter, sugar, spices and slowly stir in the coconut milk until well blended. Then, add cornstarch mixture and stir, letting it cook until bubbling gently. Stir in lime juice, remove from heat. (If you don't use it all, it'll keep in the fridge for a few days.)

To assemble, first put bed of cooked rice, then layer with spinach, the chicken strips, and cover with sauce. Fantastic!

Falafel in Pita Bread

I love falafel but when I first tried it, I was apprehensive. It's now one of my very favorite meals, good summer or winter. Give it a try, you'll be surprised, and maybe even get hooked like me. It's a staple in Middle Eastern countries, made from chickpeas (garbanzo beans). (There is falafel made from fava beans, Egyptian-style, more sour.)

Falafel mix (My favorite is the Israeli brand Osem, but Casbah makes a good one too)
Sliced fresh tomatoes
Sliced cucumbers
Green leaf lettuce leaves
Alfalfa sprouts
Tzatziki sauce or creamy dill sauce or tahini sauce
Pita bread pockets, cut in half, warmed

Mix the falafel according to the package directions. I shape this into small patties, about 2-1/2 to 3 inches in diameter. Place in frying pan with 3-4 T olive oil, and cook over medium to medium-high heat, until browned, turning as needed. This won't take very long. Drain on paper towels.

Assemble with one patty per pita half, stuffing tomatoes, cucumbers, sprouts and lettuce in with the patty. Add sauce as you like. Delicious.

Veggies and Salads

Ultimate Green Salad

>   Lots of leaf lettuce, green and red, butter
>   lettuce and/or romaine
>   Thin pear slices
>   Handful of candied walnuts (or other nuts
>   you prefer)
>   Handful of dried cranberries
>   Crumbled Gorgonzola cheese
>   Raspberries, a few or many

Toss in the quantities you want, add balsamic vinaigrette sparingly. Experiment with salads, the choices are limitless – Asian, southwestern, taco, make up your own. You can add chopped roast chicken to salads and have complete meals, just add crusty fresh bread.

Roasted Vegetables

Zucchini, sliced lengthwise (or other squashes)
Thick sliced red, yellow, orange peppers
Thick Sliced onions
Thick sliced tomatoes

Drizzle with Newman's Own Balsamic Vinaigrette dressing and marinate for an hour. Grill over coals, or roast on a cookie sheet in oven for 20 minutes at 350 degrees. This is wonderful with just about any entrée, or all by itself.

Sweet Potatoes

Sweet potatoes have gotten a bad rap, from all those Thanksgivings when you were a kid, subjected to somebody's aunt opening a can of yams and topping them with marshmallows. Put that memory away because sweet potatoes really are good, especially prepared with some creativity, and very good for you. A restaurant I know sells out of sweet potato French fries every night. Here's a couple of other choices:

Roasted Sweet Potato/Red Potato Wedges

Wash potatoes, and slice lengthwise into 3/4" or so wedges. Toss with olive oil, kosher salt and pepper until coated, and place on shall baking pan. Bake at 350 degrees for about 45 minutes. (Check they don't get too done and stick.)

Apple/Sweet Potato Bake

(While this one isn't the most calorie-conscious, it's really good.)

3 large apples, Granny Smith is good, peeled and sliced

6 large sweet potatoes, peeled, boiled, and sliced

1/2 stick butter, melted

2/3 c brown sugar

1/2 c maple syrup

1 T cinnamon

1/2 t nutmeg

1/2 t cloves

Layer the apples and sweet potato slices in a greased square or round casserole dish. Mix butter, sugar, syrup and spices and pour over the apples and potatoes. Bake uncovered for 50 minutes at 350 degrees. (You can cover for the first 30 minutes so it doesn't get too browned.) Enjoy.

Dessert

This is special occasion stuff – just to prove to everyone that you can make a fabulous dessert even though obviously you don't eat them all the time.

Raven's Cheesecake

This is evil on a plate for the waistline. But it's the ultimate cheesecake, the very best! Use a springform pan, cover the bottom and sides in aluminum foil. (I used to give these out every Christmas, and had a real assembly line. People still ask for them.)

Crust:

1-1/2 c graham cracker crumbs
3 T sugar
1 t cinnamon
1/2 stick butter, melted

Grease the pan with butter. Combine the ingredients right in the pan, mixing together with your fingers, and press into the bottom and up the sides of the pan. Chill in refrigerator while you make the filling.

Filling:

3 packages (8 oz.) cream cheese, softened to room temperature
1-1/2 c sugar
6 eggs, separated
1 pint sour cream
1/3 c flour
2 t vanilla
Juice of 1/2 lemon

Separate the egg yolks and whites. Beat cream cheese and sugar together, add egg yolks. Stir in sour cream, flour, vanilla, and lemon juice.

Beat the egg whites in separate bowl, until they hold a peak for a bit (not too stiff). Fold egg whites into cheese mixture until well blended. Carefully pour into pan.

Bake @ 350 degrees for one hour, 15 minutes. Turn off oven but let the cake cool inside for an hour. Take out and let cool for another hour before you refrigerate. If it cools too quickly, the top will crack. (It's likely to crack a little anyway, but not to worry…)

Before serving, take from pan and add a topping: I usually use either fresh sliced peaches, with a drizzle of sugar syrup, or cherry pie filling. I've seen many others, from strawberries to blueberries, your choice.

Brown Sugar Apple Cake

This recipe is originally is from Martha Stewart, but I've modified it a bit. Sinfully rich and delicious.

1 stick butter, melted
2 apples, Granny Smiths are best, peeled and sliced
1/2 t cinnamon
1 t nutmeg
1 T white sugar
1 c brown sugar
1 c flour
1 large egg, slightly beaten

Butter a loaf pan. Toss apple slices with white sugar and spices and arrange in bottom of pan. Stir together brown sugar, flour, egg and butter. It will be thick. Spoon over apples and smooth out. Bake for 40 minutes in 350 degree oven. Let cool a bit, loosen sides with knife, and turn onto plate. Slice and enjoy.

Cookbooks

At a lot of wedding showers or housewarming parties, for some reason people still get copies of The Joy of Cooking, Betty Crocker's Cookbook, or Better Homes and Gardens Cookbook. I guess this is OK if you've never even boiled an egg, or want to know how long to roast a turkey. But after I found that out, following these recipes seemed to me outdated, tiresome and in many cases, just plain wrong, with ingredients that I wouldn't use. I've never figured out why they always tell you to add salt to everything, or boil milk before adding it to things. Some of this sounds a little pioneer days and I don't think it's useful anymore.

I do love cookbooks, though – and the more pictures the better. I can't even read those closely printed no pictures at all cookbooks because I have to at least know what my efforts are supposed to look like – and besides, pictures are inspiring. I've been known to spend hours sitting in bookstores reading Italian ones especially… looking at vineyards and Tuscan farmhouses is just as wonderful as the food that's being prepared there.

Luckily, there's been a renaissance of good chefs writing good cookbooks in the last ten years, using simple recipes with fresh ingredients. Some of them have TV shows, like Gordon Ramsay (the old BBC Ramsay's Kitchen Nightmares are better than the "Hell's Kitchen" ones – watching Gordon throw down his fork in disgust swearing a blue streak while some pretentious cook turns chalk-white is priceless.)

So here's a few of my favorites. You can get great ideas from these chefs and their recipes, and don't be afraid to change them around a bit to suit your own tastes.

Gordon Ramsay – the Scots whiz kid, ex-football player turned chef, one of only three restaurateurs in the UK to have three Michelin stars. He's got DVDs, very entertaining TV shows, and some great cookbooks. Simple and great:

Gordon Ramsay Makes It Easy

Easy All Year Round

Kitchen Heaven

In the Heat of the Kitchen

Ina Garten – mentored by Martha Stewart, and she was the owner of the now closed Barefoot Contessa store. Her cookbooks started after the store closed, featuring BC recipes. Simple, but sophisticated. I've tried a lot of her recipes and they're simply wonderful.

Barefoot Contessa Cookbook

Barefoot Contessa Family Style

Barefoot Contessa in Paris

Jamie Oliver – another Brit chef with a big following who advocates fresh, simple ingredients. (Funny how that keeps showing up when you're talking about great tasting food, eh?)

The Naked Chef (He's talking about the food, not himself...)

Jamie's Kitchen

The Essential Family Cook

Jamie's Dinners

Martha Stewart – the maven herself. In my opinion, without Martha Stewart, cooking in America might still be playing in the arena of Beaver's Mom, Betty Crocker and tuna casseroles. She has been the inspiration and the creative force behind so many great cooks, restaurants, recipes and cookbooks, and still consistently comes up with new and inventive ideas.

The Martha Stewart Living Cookbook

Entertaining!

"Martha Stewart Living" Magazine

I could fill up this whole book with others, but my advice is to search some out yourself. Go to the library or the bookstore, and dig in. Especially in the Italian, Asian, French, Indian categories. My current favorite is Hamlyn's Complete Thai Cooking. What a feast for the eyes, and eventually, your taste buds. Every time I search, I find new treasures, and you will too. Don't be intimidated by chef's recipes, after all, they had to make it up in the first place, and maybe you really don't like capers. Experiment, and adapt to suit your taste.

Note: There's nothing wrong with chefs that have TV shows, i.e., Martha, Gordon, etc. I like them anyway because I like their ingredients and style. However, I'm not a fan of most of the Food Network stars or shows, although there are some good ones, check them out for yourself. I've tried a few of Rachael Ray's recipes and they're pretty good, and she obviously loves to cook, but I cannot fathom why it must be that everyone is crazed to throw food together in a hurry: "30 Minute Meals"; "Gourmet Italian in Minutes", or "Quick Thai Cooking for Dummies". This is marketing marketing and marketing. The average recipe takes under 30 minutes in the first place unless you're some kind of moron or want to try something more elaborate, which can be a lot of fun when you have lots of time. Slow down and breathe, and slow down and eat. Start enjoying your food, and the time it takes to prepare it. It'll taste better, digest better and you'll wear it better. It's like anything else, really. If you show love and respect, you'll get love and respect in return.

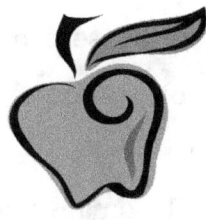

Chapter 9
In My End Is Your Beginning

The secret to weight loss is that there is no secret.

It's simply eating real food, eating less of it and getting exercise.

The other secret that's no secret is that you know this is the truth – no matter how seductive those books, magazine articles and TV ads are. We've been conditioned to think in terms of "quick" and "fast" when it comes to weight loss and this does not work. It's taken you years to develop into the person you are and body you inhabit, and it's going to take some time to change your habits and your way of thinking. I wish I could include a ticket around the world with this book, because seeing the way people eat, grow food, and live everywhere else could stimulate you immediately into changing your ways.

Instead, you're going to have to trust me and everything I've told you in these pages. It's the truth. The reason I wrote this book is because I want to tell everyone the things I've learned and what I know will work for you. I'm a medical administrator who works with the underserved. (Surprise, you thought I was an over-educated ex-showgirl with a jones for organic produce and free range chicken, didn't you?)

Every day I see more and more obese people, especially children, and frankly, it breaks my heart. Many are miserable, and a lot of the time the advice they're given falls on deaf ears – the ears of those who are least able, economically and socially, to follow it.

You, on the other hand, are different. If you bought this book, you know better, you've got choices and you just needed to find out some facts, the right stuff. You may have thought I was going to tell you that in just four or eight or twelve weeks you'd look like you lived at LA Fitness and would have J-Lo's body. Instead, you've armed yourself with information that you now have to use to get the results you want, and that takes time and effort.

Eventually, (for some of you it may be a month, for others a year) if you've been paying attention and reading this with the remembrance switch on, you will be in the shape you want to be, and wonder of wonders – smiling, bright-eyed, breathing easier, and much much happier. Once you begin – eating right, eating less and exercising will become almost second nature in no time at all.

You're going to make mistakes, indulge when and where you shouldn't, go for the cheeseburger instead of the salad, again and again. There's going to be those nights when three glasses of wine and nachos or chili fries is all you ever wanted. It happens. Don't feel guilty or stop caring about yourself, ever.

Pretty soon, you'll find you're at the supermarket, being appalled at what the people in front of you are buying, and having to stop yourself from giving them advice. In restaurants, you'll be tempted to lean over and tell someone not to order the fat-calorie-laden-deep-fried-cholesterol-inducing junk they just did, or walking up to someone buying another PlayStation for their chubby kids at Best Buy and recommend they invest in soccer lessons, hiking shoes, baseball, a trampoline or a gym membership instead. You'll control it (especially after the first or second time they tell you to drop dead or worse.).

Instead, you'll realize that you can only control you and by your example, influence the people you love, especially if you do it gently, with fresh ingredients, great seasonings, smaller portions, and love. You can do it – start tomorrow morning.

Welcome to the rest of your life.

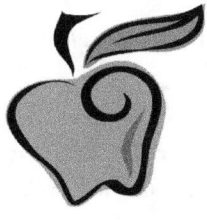

Sources

I urge you to continue on and read any or all of these books, both for pleasure and information about the food we eat, how we've gotten where we have in the processing of it, and lots of additional more scientific and agricultural information.

Brennan, Georgeanne, Breanan, Ethel, Arnold, A. *The Children's Kitchen Garden*. Tricycle Press 1997.

Freedman, Rory and Barnouin, Kim. *Skinny Bitch*. Philadelphia: Running Press, 2005.

Garten, Ina. *The Barefoot Contessa Cookbook.* Clarkson Potter 1999.

Hemenway, Toby. *Gaia's Garden.* Chelsea Green Publishing 2001.

Kingsolver, Barbara. *Animal, Vegetable, Miracle: A Year of Food Life.* Harper Collins, 2007.

Lappe, Frances Moore. *Diet for a Small Planet.* Ballantine, 1991.

Lappe, Anna and Terry, Bryant. *Grub: Ideas for an Urban Organic Kitchen.* Tarcher, 2006.

Mollison, Bill. *Introduction to Permaculture.* Tagari Publications, 1997.

Mollison, Bill. *Permaculture : A Designer's Manual.* Tagari Publications, 1997.

Morrow, Rosemary. *Earth User's Guide to Permaculture.* Simon and Schuster Australia 2000.

Nestle, Marian. *What to Eat.* North Point Press, 2007

Oliver, Jamie. *Jamie's Kitchen.* Penguin Books Ltd. 2004

Oliver, Jamie. *Jamie's Italy.* Hyperion 2006.

Planck, Nina. *Real Food: What to Eat and Why.* Bloomsbury USA 2007

Pollan, Michael. *In Defense of Food.* Penguin Press, 2008.

Pollan, Michael. *The Omnivore's Dilemma.* Penguin Press 2007.

Ramsay, Gordon. *Gordon Ramsay Makes It Easy.* Wiley, 2005.

Ramsay, Gordon. *Kitchen Heaven.* Penguin Global 2005

Schlosser, Eric. *Fast Food Nation.* Harper Perennial, 2005.

Somers, Suzanne. *Eat Great, Lose Weight.* Crown Publications, 1997.

Stewart, Martha. *The Martha Stewart Living Cookbook, the Original Classics.* Clarkson-Potter Rev. 2007.

Willett, Walter C., M.D. *Eat, Drink and Be Healthy.* Simon and Schuster Adnet Publishing Group, 2001.

Internet Sites

When you read a book like this one, at first you think, well, OK, maybe she's onto something, but really you're a bit skeptical. I mean, nobody else you know thinks the local supermarket sells poisoned apples or chemicalized junk and they aren't sick. The very best thing about the Internet is discovering there's LOTS of people out there who think like you do. You're not weird, different, or esoteric – and you've got plenty of company. Check these out:

Sustainable Table: www.sustainabletable.org – All about sustainable, organic food: what, why, and how to find it in your area, including restaurants. Root site for www.eatwellguide.org and www.themeatrix.com. Really great site. Thanks to Nina Planck.

Eat Wild: www.eatwild.com – This website is the place to find grass-fed beef, as well as fish, poultry, dairy products and the markets that sell them near you. Also great essays from Jo Robinson that tell you why this is so important.

Edible Communities: www.ediblecommunities. com – Great website that promotes fresh, locally grown food, again with connections to local links near you.

Local Harvest: www.localharvest.com. This web-site has lots of information about locally grown pro-duce, dairy products, and meat, including farmers' markets and local organizations.

Slow Food: www.Slowfoodusa.com – Slow Food is a well done site with local links and other info, but it's a trifle chi-chi and joining is a little pricey. Their heart's in the right place, though.

Center for Informed Food Choices: www.informedeating.org – This is Michele Simon's website and she's not shy about taking on the processed food industry.

Grub: www.eatgrub.org – the food revolution site with Anna Lappe and Bryant Terry.

Seeds of Change: www.seedsofchange.com – the granddaddy of organic gardening/food.

Permaculture: www.permaculture.net – start here to find a plethora of resources about permaculture gardening.